OUT LOUD

OUT LOUD

Essays on Mental Illness, Stigma and Recovery

Introduction by Ramona Dearing

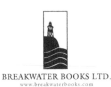

© 2010 Breakwater Books Ltd.

BREAKWATER BOOKS LTD.
www.breakwaterbooks.com

Library and Archives Canada Cataloguing in Publication

OUT LOUD : essays on mental illness, stigma and recovery / introduction by Ramona Dearing.

Includes index.
ISBN 978-1-55081-329-6

1. Mentally ill--Biography. 2. Mentally ill--Rehabilitation.
3. Mental illness. 4. Stigma (Social psychology).

RC464.A1O98 2010   616.89'00922718   C2010-901908-3

Breakwater Books Ltd. acknowledges the support of the Canada Council for the Arts which last year invested $1.3 million in the arts in Newfoundland. We acknowledge the financial support of the Government of Canada through the Canada Book Fund for our publishing activities. We acknowledge the financial support of the Government of Newfoundland and Labrador through the department of Tourism, Culture and Recreation for our publishing activities.

Printed in Canada

Cover image by Jori Baldwin
www.joribaldwin.com

 Canada Council   Conseil des Arts   Newfoundland Labrador   Canadä   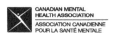 CANADIAN MENTAL HEALTH ASSOCIATION ASSOCIATION CANADIENNE POUR LA SANTÉ MENTALE
for the Arts   du Canada

TABLE OF CONTENTS

FOREWORD

The publication of *Out Loud: Essays on Mental Illness, Stigma and Recovery* is a testament to the essayists who had the courage and heart to step forward and share their stories, as well as to the determination of Breakwater Books Ltd. and the province's mental health organizations to make this book a reality. The book also speaks to the long-standing interest Breakwater has always had in social issues relevant to Newfoundland and Labrador.

Out Loud was nearly three years in the making. In fall 2007, Breakwater approached the Canadian Mental Health Association, Newfoundland and Labrador Division (CMHA-NL), with the idea of publishing a book on mental illness, stigma and recovery. CMHA-NL was enthusiastic about the project from its inception and helped Breakwater form a steering committee comprising representatives from CHANNAL; the Pottle Centre; the Schizophrenia Society of Newfoundland and Labrador; the Department of Health and Community Services, Government of Newfoundland and Labrador; the Discipline of Psychiatry, Faculty of Medicine at Memorial University; and Eastern Health. The committee met with Breakwater and CMHA-NL to discuss the overall approach — and the idea was born to let those people affected by mental illness speak for themselves.

Breakwater and CMHA-NL announced a call for essays during

Mental Health Week 2008 (May), encouraging people from all backgrounds to submit their stories.

Out Loud is the result of this process. Although we selected essays to be as inclusive as possible, this book does not intend to tell the whole story of mental illness in Newfoundland and Labrador; some aspects and illnesses are not covered. We hope, however, that this collection, coming directly from the voices of those who have been most affected, is the first step in painting a picture of the many lives that mental illness has touched. We also hope that *Out Loud* helps to dispel the negative attitudes and perceptions about mental illness that still abound.

We are pleased to launch *Out Loud* during Mental Health Week 2010. All proceeds from the sale of this book will go to CMHA-NL and to the other non-profit mental health organizations who participated in the planning process.

Thank you to all of the people who so courageously and authentically shared their stories, as well as to all of the people who came together and worked so hard to make this inspiring book a reality.

Rebecca Rose   George Skinner
Annamarie Beckel   Heather Pollett

Breakwater Books Ltd.   CMHA-NL

INTRODUCTION

Ramona Dearing, St. John's, NL

We'll call him Luke. He wore thin cotton pyjamas with a light robe over top. I remember it being more like a johnny coat. He was cold, and he was bored. He'd asked me to bring a particular book for him to read. Science fiction. His roommate slept all the time. Luke would get his clothes back as a privilege, once he showed the staff in the psychiatric unit that he could calm right down for them. They'd given him shots a couple days earlier; he'd resisted without success. He showed me the bruises. He could work up to being allowed outside for cigarette breaks. All he had to do was cooperate.

We didn't stay in his room because the roommate was sound asleep facing us, and it was strange with that dead weight in the room. We went down a long corridor — somehow I can't picture a mental hospital with short hallways — looking for a place to sit.

The place was clean and shiny and new. The orderlies and nurses said hello as they walked past. A patient paced, counting every step out loud in Arabic. People were in the art room, making things. Luke liked to spend time there drawing. I met the woman who always answered the pay phone in the hallway when I called Luke. He was a sweet boy, she said. She had straight shoulder-length hair, and she must have been somebody's grandmother. There was another young man, just a little older than Luke, who looked like he'd come over straight from the office. Clean-cut. Reliable looking. As we went by, he said hello to us quietly, politely, without smiling.

Hey, maybe you guys could be friends, I said. I remember an irrational surge of conviction, that everything would be okay with Luke if he could befriend the straitlaced guy.

We went into another room that had some chairs and an exercise bike.

Luke was glad to see me. He wanted his clothes back, and he wanted a cigarette. He was too thin. I don't remember everything we talked about. When you're visiting a member of your family like that, you talk about the big stuff, and you do anything except talk about the big stuff. The guy we'd just met was okay, but the trouble was he didn't talk much.

Luke was already running out of things to say. His brain was getting stretched, and he was tired.

So we said goodbye, and a woman on the desk pressed a button to unlock the doors so that I could leave the ward. Downstairs, at the hospital exit, signs asked people to use hand sanitizers because there was a stomach bug on the go.

It seemed so straightforward: a simple physical act to prevent a physical ailment. Plus the promise of cold air on your face after you rubbed the stuff into your hands and went out the door.

I'd never visited a psychiatric unit before that day, and it wasn't at all what I had expected. I can't say it was a cozy place, but with its big, big sunny windows it was nicer than most other wards. The patients seemed sweet, harmless. Several had relatives visiting.

Growing up, I would have told you that going to the mental hospital involved a straitjacket, a padded cell, and being left alone there for a long time. That's what we saw on television, and at the movies. And, as I understood it back then, there was only one kind of mental illness: a person was locked up for being crazy. It gave you shivers thinking about what would happen to you if you turned out that way. You'd be one of those crazy people flailing around in straitjackets in cells padded for their own protection. It was as dismissive and simplistic as that, our collective ignorance. And crushing, of course.

People with mental health problems didn't exactly go around announcing it. Families tried to contain the "shame." Jobs have been lost, friendships severed. In "Spark," *Out Loud* contributor Kim Wilton talks about the loneliness that still exists for far too many: "There are no get-well cards, flowers or visitors, only silence. Time and time again I have wished that I suffered from a 'real' disease, a disease where I would say 'I'm sick' without the stigma that inevitably follows with a mental illness."

Or as Bradley Clisshold puts it in his essay, "How do you text message the stigma of male depression?"

Prepare yourself: there are some terribly sad stories in this collection. A mother losing a fourteen-year-old to suicide. A woman believing she is giving birth to twins when in fact she's not even pregnant. Or there's Gus Russell, who always wanted to go into politics, "but now, due to the fact that I had 50+ shock treatments, my chances of living that down would be smeared all over the media genres." As Marylynne Middelkoop puts it, "One of my greatest fears is that when I die and God rolls the film reel, He will say, 'That was your life you just missed.'"

But in fact, like so many others, Marylynne's story is one of recovery. The title for her piece says it all: "Journey from darkness." And that's something that is said out loud, over and over again in this book, that things can and often do get better with the right kind of support and treatment. Here's what Janet Battcock writes: "I think it is of great importance and value to be able to talk about mental illness because that is the only way that people's fears and prejudices will be exterminated. Other people living with mental illness will be urged on by those who are able to speak out, and people who are fearful of mental illness will learn that it is an illness like any other, and can be treated and controlled."

I wish I could tell you that everything has gone great for Luke. That he found the proper counsellor and stayed with treatment and has the right kind of support in his life to rise above it all. He's been back in the hospital twice, although not for a while. He's been holding down the same job for a couple of years. But there's little happiness in his day-to-day life, and the possibility of another crisis never seems far away.

When you read this collection, remember that it probably really should include thousands more pages. Some of them would be filled with the stories people still don't feel safe sharing. Other pages would be reserved for those mired in poverty, isolation, addiction, and the many other forces that can pull people with mental illness down, compounding their health issues and effectively cutting them off from everyone else. And let us never, ever forget the unknowable number of people who have taken their own lives. Or the friends and relatives who still experience too much grief to be able to share it with others.

It took courage to submit to this book. You'll see far too much proof of the damage stigma has done. You'll also see clear evidence that having a mental illness and a fulfilling life are not mutually exclusive. There is so much generosity in these essays — people sharing some of their most intimate moments with a clear goal. And that is to reach out to others, to say out loud to them that they are not alone, and that things just may work out all right in the end. No one's maintaining it will be easy, but they are teaching by example: if they've come out the other side, the rest of us can do that, too. Because of course all of us feel the effects of mental illness, whether we're wrestling with it ourselves, or whether it affects people we care about.

The authors of *Out Loud* have helped me reach a whole new understanding of what strength really is. First of all, it takes boatloads to recognize and admit there's a problem. And then of course there's the perseverance required to make things better. Let me end with a quotation that comes from an anonymous male writer in his brief but affecting submission to *Out Loud*: "Most of my life has been pretty creepy. Today I am feeling pretty well. I married, built a house, and we live by ourselves with two cats. My advice is never quit; get referred for help. Then take this disease, take a sledgehammer and break its two knees."

A WILD, WACKY AND WONDERFUL WOMAN LIVES HERE

Janet Battcock, St. John's, NL

I have been living with mental illness all of my life. I grew up in a family in which mental illness was prevalent and we were all affected in a variety of ways. I was diagnosed in the year 2000 with cyclothymia, a type of bipolar disorder, but I am now aware that I was exhibiting symptoms of this illness as early as my teen years. This essay is about me, how mental illness makes me feel and how it affects my daily life.

The first thing I wanted to do after high school graduation was attend university. I wanted to be a primary-elementary teacher but my post-secondary schooling soon became too overwhelming to complete courses. I increasingly skipped classes and started failing courses, so I dropped out before the university had a chance to suspend me. Subsequent attempts to complete post-secondary training in a variety of fields through my young adult life have yielded pretty much the same results. But I never knew why. I convinced myself that I was dumb, even though I knew I was bright, intelligent and had thoughts and ideas that I knew other people would like to hear. I lost a great deal of self-confidence. Like most young people I worked part-time and full-time jobs but my resumé of employment experience was lengthy even at a young age. I worked many different jobs because I would have to quit jobs just mere months or even weeks after starting work. I would frequently get frustrated with people, have arguments with co-workers and become overwhelmed with small tasks.

Today I am a married woman with a six-year-old child. I don't have the privilege of being able to get up and go to a scheduled job every day. I say scheduled because I have always found volunteer work to be more flexible and therefore more suitable to my circumstances. There are days when I wish so much that I could just be *normal* and go to a job like everyone else. I don't wish for anything fancy. I have learned that steady employment is not an option for me, and it's not for lack of trying. My last paid employment, two years ago, was as a postal clerk. I didn't last through the two-week training period.

My frequent mood swings often result in the need for downtime for me. When I am hypo manic, which I call my "peak," I have more energy than normal and I am able to accomplish small tasks. I occasionally think I must be getting better because I feel so *normal*. I am nicer to people and more conversational. I enjoy being around people more often and experiencing the camaraderie of friends. But this is the time when I am at risk of making commitments that I am unlikely to be able to follow through on. Normally within a few weeks or so the hypo-manic mood takes a fairly sudden shift to mild depression, which I call my "valley." It's like all of my energy has been zapped. Then I don't feel like doing anything. Often during this downtime I am fatigued and just want to sleep all of the time. I don't want to be around other people, but if I am, there is a risk of me being easily annoyed and getting frustrated with people and things. Sometimes I will cry a lot, thinking a great deal on the things in my life that I am unhappy or disappointed about. The thing I am most unhappy about is my mental illness.

As you can imagine, having these mood swings makes it difficult to make plans. Prior to 2003 this was only a minor distraction, but since the birth of my daughter that year I have had to dig my heels in and learn how to take on the daily challenges of living with cyclothymia. In countless ways she is the reason I have had to learn how to manage my illness. I still have mood swings but I have learned they are predictable and I am using that knowledge to be pro-active. Having this knowledge has changed my life in so many ways! It doesn't change everything but it does improve the quality of life for me, my daughter and my husband. I communicate with my husband more readily by telling him when I am in a valley or on a peak. I was always the type of person who did not want to ask others for help but now I do reach out to other people. Sometimes I need an after-noon to nap or to just put my feet up and be alone. Relatives are usually more than happy to take care of my daughter for a few hours. When she is at home with me I more carefully and thoughtfully choose activities that will not further deplete my energy or frustrate me, while at the same time she does something constructive and meaningful. When I am in this valley I will avoid people and situa-tions that I know will cause me discomfort, stress and annoyance. I am satisfied with this action plan because it works for me.

There are also short periods of time between these up and down moods and I cherish these the most because this is when I truly feel normal and well. I can make good choices for myself, I can easily accomplish tasks and I can readily have conversations with people and get involved with activities. I think this is when my true nature shines through and people get to see and know the real me.

I still make plans from time to time that I don't follow through on, like baking goodies for the school fair or taking my daughter to the playground or to the beach for a picnic. I buy tickets for future events not knowing if I will want to go when the event comes up. More than once we have made family plans that had to be cancelled or changed suddenly, simply because my mood has dictated the need for change. This makes me feel guilty sometimes, thinking that I am the reason for other people's disappointment. My daughter's disappointment probably hurts me the most. I feel at times that I need to do even more for her just to make up for the times when I feel that I did not do enough.

I have had a lot of help along the way from mental health coun-sellors, a psychiatrist who has taken the time to really get to know me and strangers on the other end of a telephone line who are gentle yet frank with me. The stigma of mental illness plays less of a role in my life than it used to. I would readily admit that I had diabetes and arthritis, yet telling someone that I had a mental illness was defin-itely not an option. But since I have educated myself on mental illness and have had the opportunity to meet many other people who have learned to live with a mental illness I have been able to speak up more about my own experience with it. That is why I am able to write this essay. I think it is of great importance and value to be able to talk about mental illness because that is the only way that people's fears and prejudices will be exterminated. Other people living with mental illness will be urged on by those who are able to speak out, and people who are fearful of mental illness will learn that it is an illness like any other and can be treated and controlled.

I have been very fortunate to have a life-long partner who has been willing to live and learn with me. It is my illness, but he and my daughter have to learn to live with it, too. I can help them by helping myself. I have ditched the notion that I can do it all on my own; I am a *super woman*, but I am not Superwoman — even though I feel like it sometimes. I am learning to be true to myself while respecting the needs of my daughter, my husband and other people with whom I interact. I have a plaque in my house that greets guests as they enter and it reads: "A wild, wacky and wonderful woman lives here." People who enter my house know what they are getting — someone a little on the wild side, sometimes a little wacky, but a wonderful woman to know.

BIG BROTHER/BIG HEART

Flora Bishop, St. John's, NL

One of my earliest memories goes back to 1949 in a small Newfoundland outport. I was three years old at the time. My oldest brother, Clyde, then sixteen years old, was being brought home by a neighbour; she said he "was going to drown himself." My father, a sea captain, now disabled by a stroke, had connections and my brother was soon admitted to the mental hospital in St. John's.

Clyde had been taken out of school in grade seven and put in the fishing boat. He had seven siblings. My brother responded well to shock treatment and psychiatric medications. After his discharge from hospital he learned a trade as a machinist with the CN Railway. He needed grade ten to enter that trade but he was accepted (maybe through his father's influence) with just grade seven. He trained for five years and excelled at his job. From 1957 to 1960 he served three years in the Canadian Armed Forces. To my knowledge his mental illness was not revealed and was never an issue. In 1962, Clyde got married and had two children. He worked at the machine shop at the St. John's dockyard and loved his work. His wife was not aware that he had schizophrenia.

To backtrack, in 1954, our father died. I was seven years old at the time. There were two younger brothers ages four and five, and four older siblings who ranged in age from twelve to eighteen. Clyde was twenty and the eldest. He took on the role of father to me and many of my younger siblings. Our mother never remarried.

Clyde helped financially to keep up our house. We lived on a widow's allowance and the baby bonus. All the while he was in the army, Clyde sent money home to help us all survive and get educated.

In 1964, I was teaching school in Port Blandford. I received a call from my mother: "Clyde has had a nervous breakdown." The railway had transferred him to Port aux Basques where he had no supports. My mother and I took the train across the island. His wife, young and alone, needed help. We found Clyde behind bars at the police station. He had been found in church dusting the altar — he had a gun — he'd left home to go partridge hunting. He was psychotic and didn't know us. Seeing my loving brother behind bars will be forever imprinted on my brain. I was seventeen years old at the time. When the police arranged a helicopter, Clyde was flown to St. John's to the mental hospital. He was treated and his medications adjusted. He returned to work at the St. John's dockyard where the environment was familiar and family supports close by. Clyde received tremendous family support. He had such a kind heart, loved music, art and dance, and had a strong faith. He was very special to us all.

Family support is a major part of the puzzle when living with mental illness. I feel the emotional support is what matters most. Clyde was blessed in many ways. They say God never makes mistakes and it was certainly true when it came to his wife Mary. We helped from a distance many times but Mary was there day-in and day-out through it all. They were both very grounded in their faith and it sustained them through almost thirty-eight years of marriage. My words cannot describe Mary's devotion, patience, understanding and loving care towards my brother. It takes a very special person to support and love when the times get rough. Many times she must have felt like a single parent raising the children. I feel she was "one in a million." Very few women would or could endure the difficult times in their marriage. She always seemed to find the inner strength to face the challenges. She always embraced our family when we offered help.

In 1969, when I came home from nursing in the United States, I brought a charcoal barbecue to my brother. There were few who had barbecues at that time. I have fond memories of all our family in his backyard enjoying the weekend barbecue. He built an extra-long picnic table to seat us all. Family suppers at my mother's house for the traditional Sunday cold-plate were important events for all the family to gather. Meals and card games at Clyde's house were fun because he so loved music and dancing. In 1971, when I got married, Clyde walked me down the aisle as father-giver. We made sure that he had his place of honour in our family. Those were some of the good times. Then came the difficult times when he got sick, very sick. Because we had made such a strong bond, we never faltered. Mental illness did not define him — it was only a part of the wonderful man that he was. We visited and spent time with him in hospital. We talked with the doctors. Phone calls, cards and letters all helped to let him know how much we loved and cared for him. We supported him through every stage of his life. It seemed the loss of our father and my brother's mental illness had glued us together as a family. We all supported and helped each other.

In 1967, I received an award for psychiatric nursing at my graduation ceremony. My brother Clyde was there with most of my family. My interest in psychiatry was very strong because I wanted to understand my brother's illness and wanted to help him. Basically Clyde had inspired and motivated me. He worked and continued to be well for almost another fifteen years.

In 1978, we saw he was becoming paranoid again and as a family we rallied around him. He was admitted this time to the psychiatric unit at the Old General Hospital. He was now being diagnosed as manic depressive. Also, having back problems and having served almost thirty years with the CN Railway, he retired early with a pension. He attended his daughter's graduation ceremony at Dalhousie University in Halifax, Nova Scotia. He saw his son learn a trade as a stone mason. Again in 1994, he was admitted to the Waterford Hospital — this time being diagnosed as bipolar.

In the year 2000, at the age of sixty-six, my brother Clyde died of pancreatic cancer. His wife took care of him at home until his death per his wish. I also was with him as he took his last breath. He was like an "old angel" — so quiet and gentle. I played his favourite gospel music for him until the very end. It was such a privilege for me to be with him. At the age of twenty, with a serious mental illness, he stepped up to the plate and became a father substitute and helped us all survive and kept our family together.

From 1949 to 1994, it seems Clyde would relapse approximately every fifteen years. With the medical care and hospitalization and much loving family support, I believe my brother lived a fairly normal life. It is my wish that no one with a mental illness should ever be put in jail. When, as a society, are we going to bring mental illness out of the Dark Ages and into the light?

A COUNTRY SONG PLAYED BACKWARDS

Paula Corcoran, St. John's, NL

I stood in my small office, wearing my tan dress with buttons down the front and my favourite chocolate brown (Who doesn't love chocolate?) blazer, all topped with my most professional "How can I help you?" smile. I had prepared for this meeting. What I neglected to prepare for was the adrenaline rush. That instant of confrontation when the body's senses kick in to decide the fundamental decision between "flight or fight." The clammy hands, the flushness in my cheeks, and an ever-so-slight tremble — but he remained oblivious. In the moment it took to decide that this would NOT be a flight situation, a brief thought raced through my mind — "He doesn't know!"

"So, these bags, all made right here, hey?"

"That's right, sir! From supply purchase to final inspection and shipment. All right here."

"And this place . . . these people . . . there's something wrong with them all? Amazing!"

Breathing deep to control the tremble in my voice, unsure of the reaction to come, I replied, "Yes, sir, we ALL have a mental illness."

In the instant it took my customer to stare, mouth agape, and take an ever-so-subtle step — backwards — I had a revelation. While I spent the last three years working to harden myself to the looming daily battle against the stigmas that society has developed, I had not prepared for this. Because of my beautifully tailored clothes (purchased at a local church for 25¢ apiece), my professionally applied make-up and sophisticated hairstyle (a gift from a friend), and my somewhat educated and usually coherent speech — all coming together to land and maintain my two-year position as Customer Service Representative, this ignorant individual had no idea! I was also a [mental health] consumer. His blind remark made me feel that I was truly alone. Not "normal" enough for society, yet not quite "abnormal" to truly relate to my peers whom I considered dear friends.

Like many of my friends and fellow mental health consumers, I often find myself defending my illness. Ironically, I feel the need to convince other consumers that I do fit in — that I do belong. Despite that I "only have depression," I still suffer from an illness. While certainly not as debilitating as some of the other major psychiatric illnesses, a lot of the self-treatment, society struggles, and personal battles are very much the same.

As I recall the period in my life when I was diagnosed I often recall a discussion with a good friend during our university years. We had moved beyond country music to the rock scene and were commenting on the irrational ideas of country music.

As another lonely, broken-hearted man sang on the radio, Katie began, "We should try and figure out how to play that backwards, ya know."

Chuckling, I asked, "What? To see if there's some satanic message, like the Beatles or something?"

Shaking her head, Katie replied, "No. Did you ever listen to almost all country songs? It's always some poor guy who's lost his girl, who has no job, whose house burned down. Heck, most of 'em even lost their dog. Talk about depressing."

Following her train of thought, I added, "What a wicked song if we could reverse it. Everybody in the world would be in love, with a dream job, a mansion . . . and of course the dog would still be alive."

As we giggled as two teen girls do, we turned the dial to find a more upbeat tune, never imagining the reality in our conversation.

That's reminiscent of my past. Unlike most, I don't have a horrid childhood or years of an abusive relationship to relate my illness to; I simply woke up one morning, unable to go on. Life before that altering morning was wonderful. I had just graduated college, I had a secure career, some great friends and a supportive family, two wonderful children and, despite a recent separation from my children's father, I was involved in a terrific new relationship. And yes, I even had the dog. Life, as it seemed, was a country song played backwards. But of course, as life goes, someone hit the play button.

As I woke that Thursday morning, what little I do recall, was the overwhelming feeling of something breaking — physically feeling something internally break — and then an excessive amount of weight, making me unable even to stand straight. Having come home for a visit, my mother took one look and exclaimed, "I am making an appointment with the doctor for you — now!" Unable to speak without tears, I simply nodded my head.

As I poured out my story to my doctor — for several hours — my life was laid out and drew a scary scene. As the country song goes, all was lost. The new job — too demanding. The new relationship — over. Finances — non-existent. The kids — overwhelming. And the house — while not burnt down, had a stalker finding his way into my basement. But alas, all was not lost. Alone, and living hours from family and friends, at least I still had my dog.

At age twenty-five, I was diagnosed with depression. While my family and friends, not to mention myself, were not comfortable with a "mental problem," having expected the worst, we were all simply happy to know there was help to be had for the emotional and physical wreck that was me.

Like the months preceding my diagnosis, the initial months of therapy and treatment are sketchy at best. I do know that through the swift intervention of my family doctor and the team at the START clinic, I was quickly diagnosed and set on a journey for life as a "mental health consumer." Unlike others who would experience many emotions such as anger, or blame, I accepted and embraced my new-found identity. I also experienced an unconventional welcome when, through therapy, it was discovered I may have suffered with depression for many years, unnoticed. I could now look at myself, not as stupid, reckless or uncaring, but rather as someone suffering from untreated symptoms of a disease. Following wise words of my father — "Never say no to nothing free" — I began my quest to uncover all the supports I could, finding even the smallest opportunities to educate and enhance myself.

As life is never isolated to only one hardship, I often feel — the single mom on income support with a mental illness — that life's already given me three strikes. But most days I refuse to let that be my "out." Instead I seek. I reach out. I have found some valuable resources and some life-long friends on my journey through the "mental health" community.

While we can discuss at length the many ways our health care and government can and needs to improve, so too can we speak of the immeasurable assistance they offer. My journey to recovery has taken me quite far. I began a very passive, somewhat shy girl, at a mere twenty-five at the St. Clare's Day Treatment program through the recommendations of the START program team. Each participant with a story of their own, yet so many pains, insecurities, and struggles the same. I began to see there was room for me in this world, to have a voice, to share my thoughts. I recall one particular emotional discussion where another client, through tear-filled eyes, expressed her anger at being given this burden.

"I understand why you, single and poor, no job . . ." — like I needed to be reminded — ". . . or you, who's lost a child. But why me?"

Understanding the "single and poor" remark was not meant to be personal, my usual "who wants my opinion" self simply had something to say.

"Ms. M, I don't know why. I don't know how. Hell, I don't even know who. But I do know that someone put us all here today.

Imagine if I'd never come here and learned your feistiness, or had never been shown Ms. R's faith in God, or couldn't laugh at Mr. D trying to do tai chi."

Through the slight change in the mood, and a random chuckle, I concluded, "I don't have Ms. R's faith, but I do believe that someone is watching out for us, and *She'd* never give us more than we can handle; not without a room full of friends to help carry the load."

Astounded by my own declaration, I simply sat there and cried. And through the sniffles, I heard a reply,

"How the hell did you get so wise, and only half my age?"

That was the atmosphere of the program — a group of people brought together for many different reasons to share and comfort and teach one another through this one of many most difficult times. Naturally my time to move on arrived. Sad to say goodbye to so many easy friends, I knew our paths would one day cross again. I left to peruse other programs — Mill Lane, and PREP.

While Mill Lane, a sheltered workplace located in downtown St. John's, offered me the opportunity to re-emerge into the workforce after leaving it over a year before, it also gave me the much-needed support and accommodations to adjust to being a working, single mom. Through Mill Lane, I refined some great work skills, developed some much-needed assertiveness, and again, made some wonderful friends. When discussions around its closure surfaced, I was as downhearted as the next, but it was my much-needed push to re-enter the regular work force — which I did in stride.

In conjunction with Mill Lane, I also attended a second program. At the PREP program, efforts were made to prepare me for either a return to the workforce or to the education system. It wasn't until I returned to the workforce, and eventually to post-secondary school, that I realized how invaluable the support and knowledge of the PREP counsellors really are. Through a little assertive action and tremendous support from an individual at PREP, which has currently evolved into Community Connections, I've finally achieved one of my goals. I applied for, fought for, and received, from HRL&E, funding to return to university to complete my psychology degree. As I have learned, through the welcoming arms of my peers at CHANNAL, that although the professionals are wonderful and informed, the most effective support comes from one who can truly relate, which I intend to do upon graduation.

Our journey is never easy. The stresses of being a student and a single mom surviving on income support are never-ending. Some days I see the signs of my illness peeking at me, taunting me, looking for that vulnerable moment to creep back into my life. But I'm learning that there is no cure, but a recovery process, which includes the acceptance that the illness is not gone, but simply in remission. I'm so lucky to have been educated to recognize the signs, to be able to take an active role in maintaining my mental health. My medical team — social worker and psychologist both — assist me tremendously with that task.

And while I am still undecided as to whom, I am convinced that someone is ensuring that we are all exactly where we need to be at this precise moment. As the king of country, Garth Brooks says, "There's bound to be rough waters, and I know I'll take my falls, but with the Good Lord as my captain, I can make it through them all." Our walk through life is happening for a reason. When I think of all the wonderful people I have met, and all the knowledge I have gained, and all the struggles that have helped carve the strong, independent, passionate person I am, I sometimes, on the really good days, thank God (or someone) for deciding that depression was to be my struggle. And while country music is only inspirational played backwards, maybe listening can remind you that life isn't so bad after all . . . especially if you have a dog!

JUNE, FORGOTTEN

An interview with Judy, her only friend.

Mike Heffernan, St. John's, NL

I remember her big round glasses, and I remember her bowl-shaped black Purdy hairstyle. I remember she was tiny, like a mouse, and pretty. I can visualize her in scenes, too — walking past our bathroom, her swollen belly, her fingertips dark with ugly nicotine stains. But they are just scenes, without context. I don't remember much else because I was very young.

Twenty-five years later, my mother connected the dots for me. We sat at her kitchen table talking over a cup of tea, something we had done a thousand times. With a recorder placed between us, she was unsure whether or not she wanted to speak about this woman. I assured her I would change the names because the names were irrelevant. I wanted to know what my mother saw and heard. I wanted to know where the end had begun for her friend.

According to Statistics Canada, 29% of women are at some point assaulted by an intimate partner — a man. I now think her life, characterized by physical and emotional abuse and mental illness, was distressingly common.

W hen June and Carl split, she and the kids moved in with her mother. Talking to her, I used to think she was just crying out for help.

But as time went on she got worse and worse and was eventually hospitalized. I knew then that the person I had known was long gone.

Before I moved into the Goulds, my friend, Karen, and I decided to have a girls' night out and go for a few drinks at the old Silver Stine over on Brookfield Road. She said a friend she'd known since school would like to come along, too. Her name was June. What struck me immediately was just how nervous she was. We were sitting around having a few laughs and she was frightened to death that a guy might ask her to dance. "What will I do? What will I do?" she asked.

"I don't know, girl," I said to her. "Tell them to shag off!"

Although it seemed a bit odd, I didn't think much of it — I just figured she was extremely shy.

It would be unfair to say we were very close because we weren't; we never hung around a whole lot. We were at the same place in our lives, both young wives with kids about the same age. Once in a while, her and Carl would come over to the house for a game of cards or she'd come up for a cup of tea. Sometimes I would mind her youngsters. When my husband's grandfather died, which was a pretty hard time for us, she looked after mine.

A few things from that time stick out in my mind. One morning, I was upstairs tidying away the bed, the kids were still asleep, and I heard someone downstairs. It frightened me because I wasn't expecting company. If it was someone I knew they would've made an announcement. It turned out to be June.

For her, getting involved in ceramics with me seemed like the only social life she had. I was good friends with the one who ran the studio. A long while went by without June paying her dues and my friend decided to knock on her door. Terry dropped by to see me later that day. "My dear, you're not going to believe this. When I asked her for the money she went cracked — she went nuts. That one's a savage!"

June was such a timid person, a little tiny thing, and that came as a real shock.

Right from the start it seemed to me that everyone in her life ran the show but her: her parents, her husband, her sister. She had no say in anything. She got pregnant at a very young age and was forced into marriage. All her life had been religion, school, marriage and children. Then she was stuck at home in a community where she didn't know a soul. If you ask me, that wasn't much of a life, not much of a life at all. Then there was the religion, too. Her parents were devout Pentecostals: you can't do this, you can't do that. That's why she got married in the first place. She and Carl fought over that quite a bit, her parents wanting one thing and Carl wanting another, with June caught right in the middle.

That poor girl didn't even have a chance to live, to mature; at least, that's how I saw it.

Maybe that incident over ceramics was the start of her falling to pieces. Maybe the fact that they weren't doing the best financially, that things were going downhill for them, like missed mortgage payments and the stress of possibly losing the house, was what set her off.

It was only a few months after we moved to Torbay that her and Carl split and she moved in with her parents and the house went on the market. Mike, my husband, picked her up and brought her down for a visit. She told me everything.

Although Carl used to drink a bit, everything seemed great between him and June. From what I knew of him, he was the best kind of a guy. But what she told me was a whole different story. One time she had a black eye. I hadn't seen her for a while, a week or two, and by that time she didn't look bad at all. She told me she tripped and hit the corner of the wall. I remember that because only a few days before she was excited about being a bride's maid at her sister's wedding. Her family must've known what had happened, because if a big guy like that had punched a little scrap of a thing like her there was no way make-up could ever cover the bruises. Apparently, one time he threw a skate at her head and just missed. That'd be something to get hit in the face with, a skate. When I would visit her house

I'd see new pictures on the walls in awkward places. She put those there to cover fist holes he made when she ducked. Another thing was that before Carl left, a new family moved in next door and he accused her of having an affair with the husband. He beat her over that.

It was then that she told me her uncle had sexually abused her. Apparently, no one would believe her. The way I figured it, religious people like that just didn't want a scandal getting out.

I felt so sorry for her and thought, *Lord Jesus, what a sin.*

Because we lived on the other side of town and June didn't drive, for the next few years we didn't see much of one another. But she called. With her and Carl divorced and the house sold, she continued to live with her parents. She often told me of how she hated them, that they were controlling her, that she had to wait for them to go out before she phoned because they listened in on her conversations. I can't say whether or not that's true or if it was all in her mind.

Six or seven months later, June took an overdose. It was only then that I learned she'd been diagnosed with schizophrenia. Her mother told me.

I don't know how many trips it took going back and forth to the hospital before her parents finally had her admitted to the Waterford. I knew that she was having problems, that she was on some kind of medication to help her relax, but that's it. Even then I just assumed she'd been through a rough time of it, that her nerves were shot and she needed to be there to get her mind straightened out. But I still really didn't know just how sick June was.

For a while, we lost contact. Maybe it was because she was in the hospital and couldn't make calls. I'm not too sure. When I finally heard from her again she said she was receiving shock treatment because shock treatment made you forget things you didn't want to remember.

When June was placed in an apartment, she said she was doing pottery and taking classes through the hospital. She sounded like her old self.

Mike and I decided to invite her to dinner, figuring that maybe if she got out around people it might help her. But when she came over she was far worse than I could've ever imagined. She said she'd met a man at a dance, someone from the hospital. "I smoke now, too," she informed us. She had his pipe in her purse, hauled it out and started puffing away. I probably smoked at the time but it was all a bit much, a woman smoking a pipe.

After that, I didn't see her for some weeks.

She showed up one weekend in an awful state. She was in the hospital then and I knew something serious was going on with her. She was all zonked out of it, looked stressed and tired and everything else, was real worn down, and walked up and down the hall constantly flushing the bathroom toilet. It was then that I noticed her bleeding from beneath her dress. She was on her period but wasn't wearing anything. My husband was out somewhere and here I was with three children at home. I didn't know what to do. But she was so far gone that whatever I said she cooperated with and I got her in the tub.

I found her sister's number in her purse. "My dear," she explained, "the best thing for you to do is call the police."

That was the last thing I wanted.

Then her mother called: "Take her to the hospital. We've done everything for her we possibly can."

My God, does no one care? I asked myself.

There were a lot of empty pill bottles in her purse and I phoned the Waterford to find out how I'd be able to tell whether or not she'd taken too many. They said check the dates on the prescriptions. The most recent had only a few gone, not enough to do any real damage. Other than that, the crowd down there were bloody useless — I couldn't get any satisfaction from them. They told me the only way they could bring her in was if she got violent.

So I cleaned her up and sent her in a taxi back to her apartment downtown.

That was the last time I ever saw her.

From that point on, I started to make excuses whenever she wanted to drop by, but I can't remember hearing from her a whole lot.

Shortly thereafter, she overdosed for the second time.

That's when June's mother told me she was pregnant.

That winter it was on the news that a female patient had escaped from the Waterford and my husband's cousin, a taxi driver, told us he'd picked up a pregnant woman down there and brought her around the bay. It turned out to be June.

Years later, I met her mother at the supermarket. I asked her how everyone was doing and she said June's sister had adopted the baby. It amazed me that that little boy was healthy after all his mother had been through. In fact, they were all doing great. Brian had become a Pentecostal minister in New York working with a youth outreach program. Laura still lived in the province and had a family of her own.

She never mentioned June. It seemed to me that they never wanted her to have existed in the first place, that they had washed their hands of her. Because she still had Carl's last name, any connection to them was lost and, I guess, June forgotten.

NOBODY'S CHILD

Judy Bourne, Carbonear, NL

I am a fifty-seven-year-old woman and I have struggled with depression all of my life. Most of my life I have tried to deal with it myself. The stigma of it all kept me from seeking help, and in 1995 it became so bad I just knew I had to do something about it. Nothing in my life was right and I became so tired that I just gave up. I was like a magnet to the bed and there I didn't have to face all my hurts and fears. The hardest thing was that most people didn't understand. There were comments like, "Shake yourself," and "There is nothing wrong with you," which only made me feel guilty for being that way. There was a time when I was in my twenties I told a doctor how I felt and he made a comment like, "You should count your blessings." This did not help when it came to bringing it up to a doctor in the future.

All my troubles began when I was six years old. My dad called me in the middle of the night, and there was my mom lying dead at the foot of the stairs. Upon seeing her I became hysterical. My dad, whom she had signed out of the Waterford Hospital in St. John's, didn't exactly know how to deal with the situation. He told me to go upstairs and get a pillow and a blanket and bring those to him. I obeyed and he put the pillow under her head and covered her up. My dad was mentally ill from being in the Second World War.

He took me back to bed and left her at the bottom of the stairs.

The next morning we stepped over her and he took me to my grandmother's house. I left and I went and told a neighbour what had happened. The police came and questioned me about everything and then there were questions from the family. This happened in the middle of the night and one of the questions was "Why didn't you go for help?" It was bad enough that my mom was dead but now I felt I could have saved her. I was only following what my dad had told me; and who is a six-year-old child to question an adult or know the protocol of what to do when someone dies? All too much for a child to have to deal with. They took my dad back to the hospital and he never did come home again. I lost both my parents and I was so alone.

Autopsy showed that my mom had a diseased heart, which I found out later in life. Well, things did not get any better for me in the days to come. I went to stay with my mom's sister and a few days later a lady came to talk to her. She was from social services and they were discussing my future. Later I heard my aunt say to someone, "They won't let me adopt her because she was already adopted." My life wasn't bad enough but now I knew that my mom and dad were not my real parents. Neither were my aunts, uncles, cousins and grandparents. I somehow knew the meaning of adoption, and how I processed it all at that time is surely a mystery to me now. The only thing I know is that I wouldn't tell anyone I knew this. Maybe I thought if I told I would lose everyone. My life went on and I didn't discuss my feelings with anyone. Bedtime would be my release. I would think about it all and cry myself to sleep. I don't think there are many people out there who have cried so many tears. When I think back to my childhood I think about how strong I must have been and why, in heaven's name, I didn't crack. I think my talks with God helped me through. There were nights I would think my mom was not dead but she was just gone away. All I could think of was "Why me?" I missed her so much but could never talk about it.

I think I became a little more depressed in my teenage years. I went from an "A" student to just average. Maybe it was other things that caused the change but my focusing on things was not great. I did finish high school and went on to trades college. This was a bad year for me as my grandfather died in December, my grandmother in March, and my dad in May, and to add to it all, I was eighteen and pregnant. I got married and went on to have three wonderful children in all. There were many ups and downs and there were times I couldn't cope with life, let alone three kids. I tried so hard to be a good mother, but sometimes I would go off the deep end, break things and even tip over a table full of dishes. I guess it was the only way of venting my frustrations. I would cry excessively until I would scream and try to hurt myself. Then there would be a sense of normalcy for a period of time and it would all happen over again. My life was like a roller-coaster ride. I also had problems dealing with working outside the house. I am a super sensitive person and if anyone said anything negative to me I would well up with tears. I didn't work much as it was embarrassing for me to be like this, so home was my fortress.

In my early forties things got really bad. My adult kids started to get out on their own and I felt so hopeless and I just couldn't cope anymore. I went to my family doctor and told how I felt. When I told him that I didn't want to live anymore he was shocked and said I needed to see someone. Thank God, finally someone was listening. There was a wait for me to see a physiatrist, and the days to follow I tried to keep myself going; my husband would get me out of bed in the morning and when he left I would go right back again. I had reached rock bottom. I didn't want to see anyone or talk on the phone. I would cry for hours, and constantly thought of suicide.

Soon I got to see a lady physiatrist who listened to me and was very supportive. She started me on antidepressants and I visited her regularly. Then she referred me to a physiologist. He was excellent and worked with me for years. I also attended a couple of his support groups, which was amazing. Soon after, the lady physiatrist left for Alberta and I went to see a male physiatrist. He was excellent also. I continued to visit both for years and I could call on them anytime I was down and they would take time to listen. I just couldn't believe all this help was out there. If only I had seen someone or told someone earlier in life, maybe things would be different for me. I am still on antidepressants and I only see a physiatrist when I need to. Sometimes I want to stop the meds and then I say, "It is helping me a lot and if I had some physical disease I would have to take them." It was hard for me to bring all this up and write my story as I am trying hard to put it all behind me. I wanted to write this story as it may help others in their struggle to know there is help out there. All we have to do is ask.

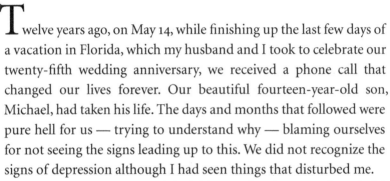

EACH DAY IS A TEST

Renee Howse, Queen's Cove, NL

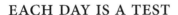

Twelve years ago, on May 14, while finishing up the last few days of a vacation in Florida, which my husband and I took to celebrate our twenty-fifth wedding anniversary, we received a phone call that changed our lives forever. Our beautiful fourteen-year-old son, Michael, had taken his life. The days and months that followed were pure hell for us — trying to understand why — blaming ourselves for not seeing the signs leading up to this. We did not recognize the signs of depression although I had seen things that disturbed me.

Michael was a wonderful child, very bright, very thoughtful, loved by all who knew him. He was respected by kids who were younger and had friends who were years older, because he was very mature at fourteen (he was 6'1" when he died). It was devastating to us when we realized he was depressed and we did not know it. Most parents with teenage children would say the signs he exhibited were typical. Since he had no outward problems such as trouble at home or at school, depression or suicide were things that never entered our thoughts. He was a great writer of stories and poems and the one thing that still bothers me concerned some poems he had written. One day I had gone through his bookbag (he had a habit of forgetting to give me letters from teachers so I would go through his bag to make sure nothing was there), and I found some of his poems. They were of a very dark nature, some even talking about suicide. I didn't confront him, as I didn't want him to think I was snooping (something I regret to this day). I did, however, mention them to his homeroom teacher who promptly dismissed them as just his way of writing. Because I was preparing for our trip at the time, I just pushed it to the back of my mind. I realize he probably would have laughed it off if I had approached him, but every day of my life I regret that I didn't mention them to him.

Over the years since Michael's death, my own sanity was an issue. I had to get help for my depression, which got me through the past ten years (I stopped the drugs over a year ago, although I still have them on hand in case I need them). Each day is a test — some are good, others bad. I attended a support group after Michael died and made friends with a woman who had attempted suicide several times before and she helped me see what Michael must have been going through.

Since Michael's death, I have little patience with people who think depression is something you bring on yourself and can stop if you choose. I have tried to make them understand that depression is not a choice (who would choose to spend their lives like that) but a disease like any other disease and must be treated as such. It is an uphill battle but one that must be pursued until the barrier is broken.

When more and more people start to understand that people with depression need understanding and support, and not criticism, then more people will talk about their problems and this will lead to fewer suicides. I tell people who criticize others who take drugs for mental health issues that I would rather have my son alive and taking drugs than not alive at all. Wouldn't any parent feel the same way! You can look at your child today and think how lucky you are that you can hug them and kiss them, hear their laughter, see them grow up. We can no longer do that with Michael. Not knowing enough about depression has robbed us of our child — don't let it do the same to you.

PUTTING IN MY SAY

Chelsea Lampe, St. John's, NL

I'm eighteen years old, and I'm originally from Nain, Labrador. I am currently residing in a homeless shelter here in St. John's. I was diagnosed with bipolar disorder in late February 2008. After years of thinking it was just clinical depression, I knew there was something more. I'll start with my first suicide attempt. I was fifteen years old. I remember feeling so unworthy, lost, hurt, confused, mad, and depressed. I thought that no one wanted me and thought I was such a burden to everything and everyone.

I never went to a counsellor or anything like that. I wasn't always comfortable talking to strangers about my problems. My friends, my family, they never understood, and neither did I. I can't imagine all the pain I put my family and friends through, let alone all the pain I was going through. Not only mentally; it also affects you physically. I dropped out of school when I was sixteen. I never did fit in. I don't think anyone does. My home life wasn't exactly perfect. I grew up on welfare and lived with siblings who were just as angry as I was about how depressing our lives were; and how I thought about my life didn't exactly help. I wanted to know why I was so mad all the time. I couldn't control these feelings, these emotions of pity, hatred, grief, and I didn't understand. I was always angry when I was younger towards the fact that I hated that I was poor. I hated how my father treated us. I hated how we moved so far away from my family to move away from my father, but no matter where I went my emotions weren't going to change. I kept denying the fact that I "needed" help. I was very stubborn about going to shrinks and what not. I've lost friends and family members to suicide and when you lose them you lose a bit of yourself, and you relate to the pain and the heartache they felt. It hurts more knowing they won't be there for you anymore.

I keep telling myself that this thing, this pain, is just temporary and everything will get better. It's only going to get better if you let it get better. Talk about how you feel, what you're thinking; it helps more than you think it does. I attempted suicide many times, thinking it was the only way out. After many years of searching and searching for this one thing I call happiness, I thought it was just a thing you find or earned like clothes or shoes or money, but I finally figured out that happiness is something you create.

It's always been a struggle to put a smile on. Even to this day it's hard; but thinking about it, there are people out there who've got it worse than me. So why waste my time being depressed? It's all about the people and environment you surround yourself with. I returned from a Youth Leadership Conference not long ago out in Ottawa, Ontario. It was so inspirational, so motivating, and spiritual. Who would have thought a conference could do that? I found out there is always someone out there to help pick you up when you're down.

I'm currently working on a support group for troubled and abused teens, but I haven't found the people here to help. I'm still searching and it's a lot of work, but I just want youth to know that there's a tonne of help out there to support you and to get you through whatever you're going through. If you are homeless, if you are being abused, if you are hurting — anything. I work at the Native Friendship Centre and when I'm feeling sad or blue I go down there. The kids just make you feel so much better. They can always make you smile and just make everything go away for that day, that hour, that minute — but in the end, it's all worth it.

I remember the first time overdosing on pills; I took 100 different painkillers. I felt so worthless just lying there in the hospital for about a month, thinking I was so worthless and no one cares about me. Then one day I had a rose delivered to me from Jens Haven Memorial School, my elementary school in my hometown. While living in Nain with my uncle, I went to the local clinic. I had talked to the nurse and explained that I wasn't sleeping and if it was possible, could I get some sleeping pills. I was having a lot of anxiety attacks and wasn't sleeping. They assumed that I was suicidal and the cops came to take me from the clinic and put me in lock-up due to the fact that they thought I was suicidal. I never had my word in and they never listened.

I was in lock-up for two nights and then they flew me out to Happy Valley-Goose Bay for my own "safety." They had me in the hospital for three weeks on suicide watch, which I found funny because I wasn't suicidal. I appreciate how they cared for me, but if they had listened to what I had to say then it wouldn't have blown up to a situation in which I did end up harming myself. I wrote a letter to the Mental Health Board office in Goose Bay. I didn't hear anything from them until a few weeks later. After leaving the hospital and returning to Nain, I attempted suicide. Everything was so stressful and it just hurt that no one let me put my word in. I just wish they had listened and didn't make assumptions. It caused me to do something I knew I didn't want to do. Then I knew I was worth more, worth more than this, and that I wanted to do something. I guess all I'm saying is that no matter how much you search for this thing called happiness, the first thing you have to do is create it. It's always going to be a struggle and I finally found out that these strangers I wouldn't talk to do help a lot, and this way it makes your mind, your head, a bit more clear and a bit more healthy. Thanks for putting my say in on what I feel.

BRIAN HAS TO GO

Anonymous

When I was very young the doctor asked my mother if there were any undo stresses in my life; he told her that I seemed to be "fretting." My mother attributed that to my overbearing and precocious older cousin who seemed to be favoured by my paternal aunts. That was the earliest indication that my brain was wired to do me harm. My father would offer his own particular brand of wisdom: "Shake it off, b'y," or "Buck up, b'y," not particularly helpful. He exercised the same brand of wisdom when it came to being near hypothermia when we went ski-dooing: "Jump around, b'y," which would be accompanied by a punch in the shoulder. Again not helpful; obvious to me now, I think it may have been wise to light up a campfire. But that's just me; don't ask me to explain where Dad's line of reasoning came from. Dad has given me so much valuable advice in life, but in freezing to death and fretting he was just plain stunned. I would be a fretter throughout life, lasting long past my scuffs over dinkies with my cousin.

I'm not sure anyone comes out of high school unscathed. Awkward, reluctant, and with a self-esteem you could fit in a pack of Sen-Sens, I persevered in spite of it. Sadly I had contemplated suicide often in that time.

In university, life would throw me a few curve balls. My best friend from high school was killed in a car accident, I struggled and failed horribly in university, and my mother lost her battle with cancer. I was twenty-four.

So there it is. My life in three paragraphs. But I'm still here; my story is still being written. I am a man in his forties profoundly affected by those early years. If youth is a time for learning, I learned failure, I learned helplessness and I learned the world was a hard brutal place. We tend to grossly underestimate the power of negative vs. positive thoughts, the sheer magnitude of the power our brains have on our lives. Like Pavlov's dog it rings the bell and I cower.

We are, after all, simply meat with minds. My particular mind likes to play tricks; it likes to tell me the world is against me, that only negative things are in my future, that I am far less capable than my fellow beings. The manifestation of my mind's control afflicts my meat-form with severe stress, anxiety, panic attacks and severe debilitating depression.

I made the active decision a few years ago to fight back. I sought the advice first of a general practitioner. She was reluctant to prescribe any sort of medication or counselling. Apparently the "shake it off" mentality extends beyond my father's scope of reason. I had to be persistent. Only I myself could look out for me now, as this was truly rock bottom.

I tried a few drugs, Paxil, Xanax, Luvox and finally — brain candy — Prozac. Prozac seemed to be my fit. I knew that studies showed that medication and counselling in combination provided the best chance for recovery so I asked to speak with a counsellor. I was told by the clinic the wait-list would be nine months.

One year later I thought they had forgotten about me. I called to check. I was still in the queue but no time was scheduled. Another month or so and I finally had a call from them. Not to schedule an appointment, mind you, but to see if I wanted to be kept on the list! Apparently even the clinic believed I could "shake it off, buck up, b'y." Holy smokes! The poor lady who had been called to handle "The List" got an earful. I got my money's worth of free counselling from the mysterious List-Keeper. I expect to see her at the Pearly Gates standing next to St. Peter. You can get into heaven — but sorry, no appointment yet.

Between the jigs and reels and after a year and a bit I get The Call. Your time has come, my son. I was to leave the waiting room and 1980s *Time* magazines and talk to an actual live person. A temp she was — down from Quebec to fill the backlog. And God love her for it, but in the few sessions before her temporary time in Newfoundland was finished she did not help. The sum of advice I took away from that was: given that I was one of the people who medicated well I should be happy enough with that. Sigh. The right combination of alcohol, Prozac and caffeine on the path to contentment.

She finished her stay and I was struck from The List. I see The List-Keeper licking the tip of a large white plume and striking a big flowing checkmark next to my name. Go directly to START, do not pass GO.

Fine enough, until old demons again found their place in my home. I struggled to find out where I could go from here. I had one last card to play. On my summer walks I pass the "Mental Health Crisis Centre." This was to be my crutch, my Hail Mary. I called to ask to speak to someone at the clinic. (The List-Keeper had been expecting this move.) I was told the clinic had now been closed and moved to the Waterford, and in case I was thinking about visiting there it was stressed that the Waterford crisis centre was pretty well exclusively reserved for people who are accompanied by the men in blue in handcuffs and shackles. I was not quite desperate enough for the criteria. Back to square one, do not pass GO.

Then . . . at long last a reprieve! My story does conclude with a glimmer of hope. A spark in a pit of coal. One last chance for Brian: an employee wellness program that led me fairly quickly to the right answers at the right time in the way of a counsellor to whom I am eternally grateful. So I sit here and type, a man with some tools to use against the demons, some understanding of them, which has greatly depleted their power. The answers were profoundly complex, yet simple. Frightening but with the weapons to fight. Dark but enlightening. With a very real sense of final hope.

Brian has to go. In order to execute a well-intentioned plan you first have to have a clearly defined goal. In my case I had to prepare for battle, but not knowing my enemy even existed makes a fight to the death rather difficult. So I needed some help to smoke him out. My counsellor led me to close my eyes as he took me on a journey to find where "he" is hiding. "You are a normal person," he tells me, "and we will work together to fight. We will find him and you will be free of his influence. You will be happy, you will be able to cope, be contented and enjoy life."

A warm feeling of calm and relaxation. I open my eyes.

"Let's go down another path now," he tells me. I close my eyes; he continues, "Your doctor doesn't care about you; he is making good money and why does he care about you? You have battled your anxiety and depression for so many years. Just when you think it is gone it returns, and you will have to live with this the rest of your life."

My heart pounds, my palms sweat, I feel defeated, alone, and unable to function in my daily life.

There he is.

The exercise was profound for me. It meant that the deepest effects of my mental illness could be induced. And if it can be induced it can be controlled. In the days following I read that this symptom, and indeed contributing cause, of my extreme low emotional state was called "negative self talk." A game of sorts my mind had created in order to wreak havoc with my well-being. I learned that this inner voice was the tip of the iceberg for how my mind had been programming itself to do me harm. This inner demon trying to do me harm was not a natural healthy part of my existence but an infection that had taken hold and had now established house for most of my forty years. Knowing this inner demon could only do harm, I was instructed to name him, find where he lives, and destroy his comfortable existence in my otherwise normal life. He is Brian.

Brian is a formidable foe. He was given birth in my childhood insecurities, grew strong during my teens and became a dominant force when my mother passed away when I was twenty-four. It was in this time Brian decided he would move in for good.

In recognizing that much of my mental strife was a learned behaviour I had to unlearn, I took this as a first step to my recovery. Unlearning something is perhaps a more monumental task than having learned it to begin with. Can we teach Pavlov's dog not to salivate when we ring the bell?

Forty plus years, three psychologists, six or seven general practitioners, Paxil, Prozac, Xanax, Luvox, countless suicidal lows, countless anxiety attacks, life's pitfalls, hills and valleys and finally a tiny flanker of what has eluded me for most of my life. Confidence, control, contentment, hope, and life.

Thanks for reading and may you enjoy all of the happiness of a contented mind and none of the demons that live therein. I hope in writing this that there can be some understanding of where things go wrong in the system and what we can all do to fix where it is broken. As for the bogeymen, they are ours to either nurture or destroy. I thank you immensely for committing something of yourselves to that battle.

THE MAN HE MIGHT HAVE BEEN

Annamarie Beckel, Kelligrews, NL

John Donne said: "No man is an island." He never knew my father.

Dad was handsome, hard-working, and intelligent, but so painfully shy and introverted that he connected with no one, not even his own wife and children. He was a blue-collar worker and farmer, a son, husband, and father who never lived more than ten miles from his birthplace. All his life Dad lived among extended family and people who had known him since childhood — and yet he had no friends. His social withdrawal was nearly complete.

His voice was gruff, as if rusty from long periods of disuse. Dad rarely spoke in sentences — only skeletal nouns and verbs — and could barely speak coherently, even to his own children. I remember being five years old and wondering, quite seriously, whether my father knew my name. I have never had a true conversation with him. How ironic that I should grow up to become a writer, a wielder of words.

It was when I sought treatment for my own depression as an adult that I realized Dad had suffered from clinical depression for decades. Yet his solitary existence was about more than depression. In today's world — if he could have been coerced into treatment — he would have been diagnosed with social anxiety disorder (aka social phobia), a mental illness characterized by an overwhelming anxiety and excessive self-consciousness in everyday social situations, as well as by a persistent, intense, and chronic fear of being watched and judged by others and being embarrassed or humiliated by your own actions.

My father's social anxiety was debilitating. Yet neither he nor my mother ever would have accepted that he was mentally ill. No one in our small farming community ever acknowledged — to his children anyway — that Dad was mentally ill, which is kind and lovely — the way that extended families and small communities protect one of their own — but also devastating — because he was never prompted to seek help and we were never allowed to acknowledge that something in our family was dreadfully wrong.

Not even his profound depression was recognized. Our childhood questions were answered by, "Oh, that's just Karl," or "He lost his mother when he was eight," as if that explained and excused every shortcoming.

He avoided every social situation he could, including time with his own family, but because everyone around us maintained the pretence that Dad was all right, we children did too. Our feelings went underground and emerged later as intense hurt and a deep sense of worthlessness. Who are you, after all, if even your own father can't love you? Later in life, we would also feel intense anger and resentment toward our father.

He was an odd, shadowy presence moving around the edges of our lives. He offered no warmth, no words of love, encouragement, or praise, no recognition for what we'd done well. As an adolescent, I thought of myself as nothing but an annoyance and a burden to my father.

He did not offer advice. He neither gave nor withheld permission — or even punishment. As my mother would say years later: "Well, at least he never beat you." A long pause. "But then again, that would have been some sort of connection, wouldn't it?"

Dad wasn't a hard drinker, a smoker, or a womanizer. He worked hard on the farm and at his job at the B. F. Goodrich plant where he worked for thirty years softening slabs of rubber for fire hoses. He spent money on no one, not even himself ... except for his gambling.

He was a compulsive gambler, an inveterate investor — and loser — in the Chicago Board of Trade, a commodities market far riskier than the New York Stock Exchange. Shortly after World War II, he'd made a profit of $50,000 — a fortune in those days. He proceeded to marry my mother, buy a new car and a new house in town — and then lose it all, except for my mother. Shortly afterwards, Mom's new father-in-law took her aside and told her to "put an end to Karl's problem."

She didn't. She couldn't. And twenty-five years later Dad's own father would exclude him from his will because my grandfather knew that any money or land he left to his oldest child would be lost.

What leads to what in the complex tangle that is untreated mental illness? How did my father's social phobia begin? Maybe there was wisdom in the words of his extended family, and it *was* the sudden death of Dad's mother when he was eight that damaged him so badly and started him on that path. Who knows? And then did his social phobia prompt him to seek relief from his anxiety and depression in the addictive thrills of gambling? Who can know that either? I can only imagine that he felt profound humiliation when he went, in his own mind, from being a "wealthy" man to a "loser." Perhaps he saw gambling as a way to overcome his own feelings of worthlessness. He may have believed that if he became wealthy again, everyone would admire and respect him: he would be worth something. No one will ever know. He never spoke of this — or of anything else — to anyone.

My mother hid his gambling — at least from his children. It was not until I was in my mid-thirties, with two young daughters of my own, that I discovered just how severe his problem really was. Mom told me that my father had put her through bankruptcy not once, but twice. He'd juggled debts on twenty to thirty different credit cards, and over the years, he'd lost hundreds of thousands of dollars.

Despite two bankruptcies and fifty-two years of cajoling and admonishing from Mom, Dad never stopped gambling until, at age eighty-three, he suffered a stroke and could no longer make sense of numbers. My mother's story of how she got him released from the hospital became fodder for family folklore — ironic humour of the darkest kind. At a meeting of the professionals involved in treating my father, his primary physician said that he thought Dad was ready to be released. The psychologist immediately objected: "This man cannot be released yet. He's uncommunicative, hostile, and incoherent." At that point, Mom interrupted: "That's not the stroke. This man has *always* been uncommunicative, hostile, and incoherent." And so Dad was released.

My father never meant to hurt anyone. He wasn't a bad man; he was simply damaged himself and oblivious to the damage he left in his wake. And although my mother could be considered his enabler, she is also the heroine of this story. Were it not for her, Dad would have been the old cranky hermit living out on the farm by himself.

Mom is also a heroine because she "normalized" our lives. She wouldn't leave her marriage — she was of the generation who "just didn't do that" — but neither would she accede to our father's dour moroseness, social withdrawal, and addiction. She was enormously courageous. She gave us love, attention, guidance, and laughter.

Our father had no friends; she had many. We celebrated every holiday — whether our father participated or not. We took summer vacations — whether our father came along or not. She became both mother and father to us, and even though money was always tight and we lived in a rundown house on a small farm owned by my father's step-mother (Mom and Dad would live in that house for more than forty-five years), we wanted for nothing important. I believe she saved all three of us from severe mental illness of our own.

When I was ten, Mom returned to work full-time as a physical therapist, training she had received in the army during World War II. Because of the marvellously quirky marital property laws in Ohio — for which I will always be grateful — she was able to bank "her" money in such a way that Dad could not access her accounts: her money could not be used to cover his debts. Single-handedly, she saved enough to put her two sons and her daughter through university debt-free. In later years, she even managed to save substantial sums to leave for the education of each of her seven grandchildren.

She gave us our lives and our freedom. She taught us how to be strong. She taught us to dream. She taught us what it means to love.

Two years after my mother's death, my father died at age ninety: an island within a sea of people who would have loved him . . . if only he'd been able to open his wounded heart and let it be healed.

My mother's legacy is one of faith, hope, and love. My father's legacy is one of damage: depression, cynicism, and feelings of worthlessness. Sometimes I curse that legacy, but just as often I weep for the father he might have been, for the man he could have become.

WEALTHIER NOW THAN BILL GATES

Anonymous

This letter is only a short summary. My age now is my handicap to write. I am eighty-eight years old now and it's telling in my writing.

I am a survivor of mental illness. The first time I knew there was a condition called being nervous was when I was in my early twenties. I am now two years from ninety years old.

Then I was totally ignorant of such a sickness. I was in an extremely stressful situation, married, living in an extremely dysfunctional family and surviving on, as far as I can remember, $27 a month for four of us, including the baby. I had to be married, and worse still, my husband's aunt spent these few dollars. I thought unwisely. I lived all my life in hiding. Kept the extreme condition to myself. I would not disclose all of this to my mother because she worried.

That was 1940-41. The war was on; the world was struggling from the financial depression of the thirties. I went to work drying fish. The mentally disturbed owner at the job suddenly hit me across my back with a dried fish. I landed in the hospital with a six-week fever. I only relate this incident because the fever must have destroyed some nerve tissue; my spine and top of my head felt like they were on fire. It seems the shock put me in the hospital. A child in a hysterical condition got out of bed and came over to where my bed was. There was no nurse on the ward at the time. Because of the condition I was in, I reacted to the shock of the child, and when they took my temperature that evening it was down for the first time.

Now the rest of my life has been dramatic all the way. It would take a great many books to tell. I am struggling with damaged nerves, added to the mental condition first caused when I was fourteen and a half. I was sexually abused at fourteen and a half by a relative (an adult), and sworn to secrecy. When the doctor told me I had a nervous condition, I haunted the libraries to learn what I was confronted with because it has destroyed my basic pattern. I had to learn how to crawl out of it, and I am still learning: learning to work handicapped, acting normal, because of the social (seems world-wide) stigma.

I understand all of you who suffer, and I empathize with you. I cannot empathize with the world. It seems they are all as ignorant as I was. A few years before I went to Montreal, I had outpatient insulin shocks, and the social worker found me a job as a nursing assistant at the Waterford. I worked there six months and saw the patients' behaviour. When I came among the normal people I saw in them all the same traits of behaviour, but they do not know it. People everywhere are not 100% normal. How can I feel, logically, why I am as normal now as I am? Right medication has helped a great deal, and therapy. Recovery came by reading and writing and prayer. Write out what you are thinking and it will reveal a great deal. Keep writing.

I am wealthier now than Bill Gates, only partly because I was always too exhausted to spend my minimum pay salaries. The greater wealth is something else. The vast majority of earth has a centre that aches with emptiness. During my years with mental illness I suffered a thousand hells. That too is not understood by the normal. Now I have a supernatural spiritual wealth that I would suffer all over again what was so great an agony of pain. Now I have fellowship with the great Creator. He is closer than the breath I breathe. Here again in this realm, there are counterfeits of new age and other counterfeits too numerous to mention, and media. I walk with a throng down through the ages, who know what I'm saying, or have known while some were on this side of eternity. Because of this I have insights that come from the Holy Spirit of God, the Creator, who lighted my way, step by step, miracle by miracle, out of mental illness.

Lastly, I know now God created sex to be so holy and pure, so beautiful if experienced between a man and wife and family as the Creator formed it, and showed the way; but we also have a spiritual enemy who is so diabolically evil and destructive. He's the one who caused mental illness and all the ills. He is the author of lies and stigma and ignorance. But God's word says there will be an end to him and his works.

JOURNEY FROM DARKNESS

Marylynne Middelkoop, St. John's, NL

Picture, please, the front door of a house. It is a dark-stained wood with a weathered patina and tarnished brass doorknob. It could be the entry to anyone's house — yours, mine, that odd recluse who lives down the street. The doorbell rings. Once. Twice. No one answers.

A hushed voice from inside begins to speak and we are privy to the home-owner's thoughts and feelings. Afraid to answer the door, she has hidden so she won't be seen. She's not sure if it's safe to come out. What if someone is still there? Her fear, loneliness, and despair are tangible as she becomes more and more despondent.

A folded newspaper hits the front door and lands on the porch. You see other papers lying there as the camera pulls back and widens your view. A voice-over makes a closing statement to the effect that if you or anyone you know feels like this woman, it may be a sign of depression or other mental illness. Confidential, professional help is available for you via the displayed phone number.

I was in my early teens when this commercial aired and, almost four decades later, I still remember my mixed feelings of dread and relief upon viewing it. I identified with so much of what the woman was saying — the fear of answering the door, the hiding until who-ever it was went away, the weighty feeling of hopelessness that made it difficult to think or even speak. I was surprised and relieved to know there were others who felt the way I did, yet I felt more alone than ever.

I have a long history of abuse and have struggled with feelings of inferiority, hopelessness, and rage much of my life. In my experience, abuse taught me that I was worthless and filthy — a throw-away. Repeated abuse — not by the same person necessarily, but by several different people — validated this.

As a child, I suffered from recurrent, screaming nightmares, and was afraid to be alone in my darkened room. Growing up, I had one friend. When we were together, our world was as big and wonderful as our imaginations would allow. For six years I was confident, free, and relatively happy. She moved away when I was ten and my life was never the same.

In my teenage years, I didn't seem to fit in anywhere; loneliness was the one constant I could count on. I spent a lot of time in my room, allowing my imagination to take me places I didn't necessarily want it to. I still remember the terror I felt the afternoon I looked in my mirror and did not recognize the reflection staring back at me.

I was afraid to look directly at people. I would cross the street before they got too close so that when we passed, there would be a road between us. Our basement stairs were open in the back and I was convinced something horrible lived under them, waiting to grab me and drag me into its lair. I dreaded going into the basement. Reason told me there was nothing under the stairs, yet I always ran back up them as if my very life were hanging in the balance. Once "safe" in the kitchen, I struggled to slow my heart rate and ease the grip of panic that squeezed the breath out of me.

These were burdens I carried alone. I dared not speak of them to anyone.

Driven by a need to be perfect, I believed if anyone found out what I was *really* like, they would be repulsed, and I would be alone forever. I felt I needed to live an exemplary life so my nasty little secret would remain just that. Living this way consumes a tremendous amount of energy and cannot be sustained forever. Eventually, something snaps.

I entered the mental health care system eleven years ago at age thirty-nine. My methods of coping didn't work anymore. My thoughts and behaviour were becoming erratic and frightening — both to me and to my family. I was prescribed medication for depression and had bi-weekly sessions with my psychiatrist. The goal at this time was survival, plain and simple.

My husband wanted assurances that I would get better, but my doctor couldn't provide that guarantee. The best we could hope for, she said, was that I regain a level of functionality and learn to live within my limitations.

After several months on medication and seeing no real improvement, I felt pressured to stop taking it. Eventually, I began to doubt its merit as well. My doctor, once assured I was making an informed decision, gave me a schedule to follow to wean me off the drug. Within days of my last dose, I experienced the deepest, most intense plunge into blackness I'd ever had. Even though my doctor had assured me I could come back to see her if I experienced any problems, I did not return. I still don't know why. I suffered through two years of debilitating depression and suicidal thoughts before finally calling and asking — no, begging — to be taken back.

I returned to the mental health care system in worse shape than when I had left it, yet in many ways I was stronger, determined to submit to my doctor's treatment plan no matter what anyone said.

I was put on different medications and had regular check-ins with my doctor. She referred me to a psychologist in the private sector until I could be taken on by one within the system. The wait was lengthy; I chose to remain with my original psychologist. When my insurance provision ran out, he referred me to a social worker in the family violence department of the health care system where more resources would be available to me than what he alone could provide. I still see him for monthly "tune-ups."

Trust is very difficult for me. It has taken several years with the same therapists to get to the place where I can talk about certain issues. My entire journey has been one of learning and growth, much like peeling an onion layer by layer. With the removal of each layer, tears come as I learn more about myself and the behaviour that resulted from the abuse I endured.

What I have learned in this process is that "normal" really is just a setting on your dryer. One person may view another's behaviour as self-destructive and deem it deviant or even crazy, when, in actual fact, it is simply a normal response to an *ab*normal past. The coping methods of a traumatized person will naturally be frightening for one who has never experienced abuse or trauma. I've decided "normal" is a relative term, defined by culture, experience, and temperament.

One of my greatest fears is that when I die and God rolls the film reel, He will say, "That was your life you just missed." It has been said that, until the pain of staying the same is greater than the fear of change, we will never change. I reached that point two years ago. I was tired of simply existing, of going through the motions while waiting to die. Even though I was willing to do anything to put my depression and PTSD behind me, I felt extremely vulnerable because I would be changing what I had known most of my life, what I had become comfortable, albeit miserable, living with. Frightened, I began to question what lay ahead.

What if nothing got better? What if, after all was said and done, this was as good as it got? What if life was really just one big, cruel joke? I couldn't bear that possibility, did not want to continue living if that were the case. My social worker assured me there was hope for a better life beyond my depression. I chose to let her hold that hope for me until I could embrace it myself.

My recovery thus far has been a long, slow, and sometimes painful process; I'm thankful for the coaching and encouragement I get every step of the way. I may not recover fully, and I'm okay with that. My goal is to grow stronger through acquiring knowledge and insight and to learn to accept things the way they are rather than obsess about how far I am from my idealized perception of happy, healthy and normal.

I still have set-backs — times when, for the life of me, I cannot remember what the point to anything is, times when I fear I will be completely swallowed up by the blackness that pursues me. This is when my support system of mental health professionals and friends is most valuable as I remember their words and choose to believe them. Yes, there is hope for me. Yes, I am worth the effort. Yes, this episode will pass, just as all previous ones have.

Through it all, I've begun to recognize several key elements to my ongoing recovery. Vulnerability has been a necessity. I continually need to break down the walls I erect to keep pain out. In trying to protect myself from further hurt, I effectively seal myself off from anything good as well. I need relationships with others — professional or otherwise — and must learn to trust them and accept their help.

Education is equally vital. I try to learn as much as I can about my particular problems and why I react the way I do to certain triggers and stressors. With the diverse and often-times contradictory information available on the Internet, I look to my health care providers for help in discerning what is valid and what is not.

Assigning purpose to my pain is an ongoing focus. It is important for me to know that what I have endured has not been pointless; if I am able to help just one other person, my past, and the effects of it, will be a little easier to live with. To that end, I've become a self-proclaimed mental health advocate, speaking up when people make uninformed judgments or comments about those with mental illness. I also help facilitate a women's abuse recovery group; there is power in knowing we are not alone in our experiences or our pain.

Above all, my recovery cannot be separated from my Christian faith. A friend and mentor who has walked this journey with me for several years introduced me anew to the God who created me and who loves me. Through her example and teaching, I now understand that real love is not earned, but freely given, and that my identity and value are rooted in who I am as one of God's children, not by what I do, or by what was done to me. I am a product of my past, but my past does not define me. My diagnoses are of little import, serving only to let me know what I am dealing with and need to educate myself in. Again, I am not defined by them.

As I begin to trust God with more and more aspects of my life, I discover He is fully trustworthy. I am confident that whatever my future holds, He will be there, providing for my every need.

When I feel I have no hope, He will connect me with someone who will hold hope for me. When I feel out of control, He will provide someone who will listen and not judge, guide and not push — someone who will give me coping tools and teach me how to use them. When my world is shaken and I lose sight of what is real, He will send someone who will pray with me, and He Himself will calm the storm and turn me back towards truth.

SHATTERED DREAMS AND BROKEN HEARTS

Christina S. Y. Keough, Bonavista Bay, NL

This story that I am about to type is a very painful one. I am a mother of two children who today are nineteen and seventeen years old. You see, I am a mother who has spent all of her life sick. You see, I was born with a bad heart which required surgery when I was a baby and I also have seizures. Also, as a baby, I suffered a stroke. As I became older my left lung got bad and I had to have half of it removed. As I grew into an adult, I was always advised not to have a child. But me being me, I went against the odds and had not one but two healthy children. When my children were eight and ten years old I suffered from another stroke. This one left me paralyzed from my hip down to my knee. Within six months I realized I could no longer read or write and I lost all of my learning. So here I was, I could no longer read, write or walk, and at that time I could no longer remember giving birth to my children.

I had lost all memory of my children for a while. It was as if I was hurting strangers yet in the meantime they were my own children — my flesh and blood. I had no memory of them and it was placing a hard strain on all of us, especially my marriage. According to doctors, I was very sick and I had given up to die. My parents then had papers drawn up stating that the children were to remain with their mother up until their mother's death. And if anything were to happen to me they were to get full custody, but the children were to remain with me. We went to court in 1999 and won our case on June 29, 1999, about a month before I was diagnosed under the care of a doctor.

My mother wanted me to see someone, but I didn't want to because deep down inside I knew, once you go in under mental health, you are looked upon differently, but through great persuasion I later went. My doctor later diagnosed me with post-traumatic stress disorder. I remained under his care for two months. And then, after being home only a month, I was admitted back there again. It was then that I began to realize what I had been hiding for years. While under the care of my doctor, I unlocked a part of my life that I had been hiding, and that was my abuse and rape as a child.

I will admit to this very day it hurts me deeply to know what has been done to me as a little girl up until I was almost thirty-seven. I spend a lot of time overcoming it by typing in my book. At first it seemed like the book was not so hard, but as time went by and when I lost my children in November of 2001, it unlocked a part of my life that I had dreaded and feared for years. And when it unlocked this part of my life I finally decided to do something about it. And do you know something? I did in January of 2002. And here I am today, at the age of forty-six, still waiting. The sad part of all of this is when I finally came forward they did nothing. To this very day I still have nightmares and trouble coping. I keep asking myself, "How could this happen? And why me?" I guess that is something I'll never know.

Throughout all of this, tragedy struck home once again. Here I was, a mother of two who could not read or write, and I was faced with court papers that to this day I still can't understand. Because here I was, talking to a lawyer who had been my lawyer only a few months earlier. And little did I know that I was being taken advantage of. Here was a woman who could not walk or read or write. Yet false promises were made. Promises that would eventually come back to haunt me. And then within ten months a mother who had loved her children was denied, and within 48 hours I lost custody of my children. The sad part of all of this is that they could not find me an unfit mother. They used my seizure drugs, along with the fact that I had gone in under mental health. You know they say their system is great, but over the years the system has failed me in many ways. I no longer trust the system. I spend most of my spare time typing in my book, a book that is mostly about our system and one woman's fight to seek justice for herself and her children.

Since I began my book in 1999 I have learned many things. You can't judge a book by its cover, just as you can't judge a person who has gone in under mental health. Yet it is supposed to be there to help you. But when push comes to shove the word mental is used more than what it stands for. Not all people who go in under mental health are crazy, yet we are looked upon that way. It makes you stop and wonder. I know it does me. I hope someday to give my book to my children. A book that explains everything about what their mother has gone through since she's been hospitalized. And how one mother fought right from the beginning. I call my book *Shattered Dreams and Broken Hearts* because every dream I ever had of being with my children got shattered that year, and hearts got broken when three people who were once a loving family were no more. Just because a mother got help that is provided for people going through hard times.

I guess you could say I'm lucky in one way. The book I am writing has helped me deal with a lot of things in my life. I am happy to say I am on no medicine for my post-traumatic stress disorder. There are days when I get down I turn to the computer, and I go into my book and write about each day and how I am coping. I will admit it is not an easy process. And we all need help from time to time. I found today hard, but by the time I finished this I felt a little better. And there are times that I have more bad days than good. I am proud to say that I have not been hospitalized since December of 1999, and then in July of 2000 I remarried, and each and every day I thank God for giving me the gift to read and write and to be able to walk again. And I also thank him for the kind support and help of others who were there for me when I needed them the most.

A TRIBUTE TO JIM FARDY, THE FOUNDER OF CHANNAL

Steve O'Brien, Roger Baggs & Moyra Buchan,
Deer Lake & St. John's, NL

Jim Fardy was a close friend, the driving force and one of the founding members of CHANNAL (Consumers' Health Awareness Network Newfoundland And Labrador), a provincial organization that exists to build and strengthen a self-help network among individuals who live with mental health issues. CHANNAL's aim is to combat isolation for those living with mental illness, to provide a forum for mental health consumers' concerns, to educate the public on issues relevant to mental health consumers and to offer advocacy, as well as social and emotional support to mental health consumer/survivors/ex-patients.

Jim was a practicing lawyer who had developed a mental illness in his early thirties. In 1989, the national office of the Canadian Mental Health Association (CMHA) was sponsoring the development of consumer/survivor/ex-patient groups across the country and had a consumer networker on staff, Julie Flatt. Prior to a planned visit by Julie to St. John's in October of 1989, Jim volunteered to organize a meeting for her to speak with people with mental health issues and illnesses. He called or visited all the mental health programs both in hospitals and in the community, and invited people to attend. There were about fifteen at that initial meeting. Julie informed the group about consumer/survivor/ex-mental health patient initiatives in other provinces and the kind of things they were doing. At that time, self-help was not even a blip on the radar in Newfoundland and Labrador. Those in attendance were impressed and excited and decided to meet every second Saturday afternoon in a location made available by the local CMHA. Attendance grew regularly and by Christmas of that year, the group decided to meet on a weekly basis. By the spring of 1990, numbers were over forty.

One of the key factors in the growth of CHANNAL during those months between October of 1989 and April of 1990 was Jim Fardy himself. He used to phone everybody between meetings, chat with them, and encourage their involvement. He facilitated meetings beautifully, making sure that everybody had a chance to talk (only if they wanted), and also involved everyone in deciding the name and logo of the group. (The name CHANNAL became official in April of 1990.) Jim's style of leadership was to build on consensus — he didn't believe a self-help group would survive and prosper without strong involvement by its members. In May of 1990, the first CHANNAL provincial conference was held in St. John's with about seventy people attending from all over the province. In the fall of that year, the Newfoundland and Labrador Division of CMHA received $95,000 from Health Canada to start and develop consumer/ survivor/ex-patient groups across the province. This allowed a number of volunteers to receive training and to have their expenses covered in visiting a number of locations in order to hold presentations and to generally "spread the word" about CHANNAL.

It is no exaggeration to say that CHANNAL wouldn't have gotten off the ground without Jim Fardy. All who knew him respected him, and everybody felt equal. One success story in which Jim played an instrumental role was to help an individual who had been out of the workforce for a number of years. He provided a reference and set up an interview for the person. At the time, employment opportunities for individuals with mental illness were not widespread. As a result of Jim's actions, and his caring and concern, this person found a job and kept it. Jim provided an enormous amount of support to the group to help make people comfortable, including offering rides to

CHANNAL meetings for those who needed them. Participants who would normally have been reluctant to leave their homes because of the symptoms of mental illness were now able to attend thanks to Jim's compassion and generosity. Jim also shared the costs with CMHA for purchasing snacks. There was a break room off the meeting area, where, over coffee and donuts, people got to know each other better. These informal conversations helped to break the ice and make people feel more at ease when sharing their stories with strangers. After a few meetings, "strangers" became "friends," and the group was off and running.

As CHANNAL grew, Jim took on more and more volunteer roles, both within CMHA and the newly formed National Network of Mental Health (an umbrella group linking all the provincial mental health consumer/survivor self-help organizations). By 1993, the demands on his time and involvement were becoming too stressful and his own health was suffering. Never one to seek the spotlight, Jim preferred a much lower media profile, opting to let other CHANNAL members conduct media interviews and attend public events in his place. By the end of that year, he decided to wind down his activities from CHANNAL. He still kept in touch with many of us, and always maintained a keen interest in the consumer movement.

Complications from kidney cancer led to Jim's sudden and un-expected death in October of 2007 at the age of fifty-four. In Jim's memory, CHANNAL introduced a Volunteer of the Year Award. Jim Fardy will always be remembered as a kind person, a leader, a friend and mentor in the self-help movement for mental health consumers/survivors in our province.

THE ITSY BITSY SPIDER

Heather Y. Boone, Red Deer, AB

> *The itsy bitsy spider went up the water spout.*
> *Down came the rain and washed the spider out.*
> *Out came the sun and dried up all the rain*
> *And the itsy bitsy spider went up the spout again.*

My three-month-old son loves it when I sing to him about the itsy bitsy spider that climbed up the water spout. I can't even get through the first few lines of the song before his lips curl up in a toothless smile. I never realized how ironic his love for this song was until my mother heard me singing it to him. "Isn't it funny," she said to me, "that you used to be so afraid of spiders and he just loves that song?" As I contemplated the irony in my son's song preferences, I began to reflect on how far from humorous my arachnophobia had been.

With an undergraduate degree in psychology, I had been trying to psychoanalyze my fear of spiders for years. I postulated that the fear began when I was trapped in a bathroom with a rather large spider on a high school trip to Australia. It was sometime after this incident that my dislike of arachnids changed to become an irrational fear. I later learned in university that the difference between a fear and a phobia was that a phobia would significantly impact an individual's life. It didn't take much reflection to realize that I had more than a simple fear of spiders.

I always thought that Newfoundland was paradise for the eight-legged menaces. Every bench, every patio, and every window seemed to be donned with the sparkling threads of the creepy crawlers. While most people welcomed the promise of warmer weather with the coming of spring, I would mourn the end of winter and months of relaxation. For me, spring brought anxiety into my life. The thought of spiders' nests bursting with movement would bring shivers to my spine. I dreaded such images. And as a result, I began to engage in avoidance activities to address my fear. It is a common behaviour for individuals with phobias to avoid the stimulus they fear most. However, with Newfoundland's abundance of spiders, this was nearly impossible. So I had to be more creative with my avoidance strategies.

First, I started to avoid sitting where spiders might be lurking. I refused to sit on picnic tables, lawn chairs or even the steps of a patio. In order to avoid the stigma of being crazy, I would always inform friends that I would rather stand then sit. It was rarely questioned. Unfortunately, with time, my avoidance strategies became more numerous and complicated. I soon began wearing clothing with hoods to avoid potential falling spiders from doorways. Eventually I had to wear mittens to take mail out of the mailbox or to turn a doorknob. Even in mid-summer I was walking around like I was prepared for a snowstorm. I began to collect cans of spider-killing Raid under my kitchen counter, and at the height of my avoidance strategies, I began to carry a can with me at all times. I'd be heading to the university for class with textbooks, notebooks and Raid.

I have always found that people didn't take me seriously when I said I was afraid of spiders. So many people say they're afraid but really only have a strong dislike for the arachnids. And when friends and family began to take notice of my avoidance strategies, they responded by telling me that I was being "foolish" or "silly" and that I should "get over it." It was frustrating because I so desperately needed support to combat this phobia, but I was given very little. It always seemed to me that phobias were so rarely distinguished from simple fears and were rarely understood.

The turning point for me came when I discovered a spider on the ceiling of my home. Although I had made such discoveries before, there was always someone there to rescue me — someone who could slay the beast and alleviate the fair maiden's distress. But at this particular time, I was alone. And there, high in the corner, sat my nemesis. He was large by any Newfoundland standard — a plump abdomen with eight long legs slowly moving. And I was alone. There was no hero to rescue me. So I did what any fair maiden would do in such a desperate situation — I called my father.

At this time, my father was at work. And his workplace was at least twenty minutes away. When I asked him to leave work and drive across St. John's to kill a spider in my house, I don't think he took me seriously. But I was very serious. I think I would have given up food for a week to pay someone to come and kill that spider for me. But my father didn't understand how advanced my fear of spiders had become, and he clearly indicated that he would not be coming to my rescue.

With my eyes never leaving the spider, I tried to phone numerous friends and family members, only to be met with answering machines or ridicule. As I watched the spider (who hadn't moved an inch), I burst into tears of frustration. I was frustrated that I was so scared of such a tiny creature. But I was also frustrated because I didn't know what to do. I couldn't leave the spider there, because I knew it would crawl to some nook or cranny in my apartment and surprise me with its presence at a later date. I had to get rid of it before it started to move.

So with tears rolling down my cheeks, I dressed up in my winter's garb — everything from a hooded coat, to ski goggles and mittens. I left no piece of skin exposed. Then, with a can of Raid in each hand, and my heart beating ferociously, I moved in for the kill. One shot from the spray can, and the beast was slain. And then I stood there, and realized in that moment as the spider fell to the floor and wriggled to its death, that I needed to get professional help.

By the time I realized I had to do something about my arachnophobia, a new challenge emerged. It took me months to finally make an appointment to see a therapist because of fear. It was not only the fear of spiders that was plaguing me, but the fear of the negativity society often directs towards those who receive counselling. I was afraid of someone finding out that I was seeing a therapist. After all, I didn't want to be labelled as "crazy" or "nuts." Although I was studying psychology at Memorial University, I still had trouble escaping the stigma attached to the therapeutic process. Overcoming that stigma, however, allowed me to take charge of my life.

When I eventually found myself sitting across a room from a therapist, I had finally convinced myself that I had to battle this phobia or it was going to consume my life. I was ready for just about anything! But when the therapist suggested "systematic desensitization" I didn't realize what battling this phobia would entail.

Systematic desensitization is a process in which the patient is gradually exposed to different anxiety-causing stimuli through a series of steps. In order to adequately address the anxiety, the therapist will teach the patient a variety of relaxation techniques (i.e. deep breathing). As part of this process, I first had to create a list of all of the anxiety-provoking situations I could think of that involved spiders. This was not a difficult assignment! At this point I couldn't even think about spiders without it causing some anxiety. By completing this list I was able to recognize what I was most afraid of. On the bottom of my list, I had written that seeing a spider on television or in a book caused minor anxiety. Seeing a spider outdoors in a web was listed as moderately anxiety provoking. At the top of my list, producing the greatest anxiety, was being next to a live tarantula. Even the thought of this situation caused me some minor discomfort. I actively avoided what I termed "arachnid avenue" in any pet store. The thought of one of those large and hairy creatures within a few feet of me caused my skin to crawl. I even had difficulty watching any reality television show that used tarantulas in their programs for different competitions. A friend once asked me if I would be able to hold a tarantula for a million dollars. Sadly, I would have seen such rich hopes evaporate in a cloud of fear.

The therapist had to explain to me that, in order to overcome my fear, I would eventually have to face what I feared the most, and come face to face with a live tarantula. My face turned white at that moment of revelation. I felt nauseated and weak as the blood drained from my head. I will never forget that feeling. I knew how challenging this would be for me, but I also knew how important it was that I meet that challenge. So with hesitation, I told the therapist that I was ready for whatever needed to be done. I was signing a contract within myself to change a part of me that I needed and wanted to change.

Over several counselling sessions, I observed my fear of spiders gradually diminish. With the relaxation techniques the therapist taught me, I was able to slowly overcome my fear. Eventually, images of spiders no longer bothered me, and I was even killing small arachnids around my home. As I battled this phobia in the counselling office, I also noticed that my self-esteem and my overall outlook on life were becoming increasingly positive. I was feeling better about myself, and I was elated with my accomplishments. In retrospect, I find it hard to believe that I was so hesitant to seek out such life-altering help. After a dozen sessions with the therapist, I was finally mentally prepared for graduation day.

Graduation day. For the graduate it is often the end result of years of hard work, and hopefully the start of a new chapter in one's life. While most graduates have to walk across a stage and receive a piece of paper to commemorate this event, I was given no such memento. However, my last session in counselling will be an experience that I will never forget.

In this final session, my therapist brought me to a pet store where he had arranged a meeting for me with an arachnid enthusiast.

This enthusiast was a young man named Daniel who worked in the pet store and spent most of his time in "arachnid avenue." He had two pet tarantulas at home, and he had brought along a friend for our meeting. His friend was of the eight-legged variety and was affectionately named "Rosa."

Rosa, a Rose tarantula, was small in comparison to many tarantulas. I remember the therapist calling her "cute" when I first met Daniel and Rosa. I recall thinking that puppies and kittens are cute, not tarantulas. Daniel and the therapist brought me to a meeting room within the pet store that is designed as a place where customers can have some private time with animals in the store prior to adoption. Inside the room there was a large table. My therapist and Daniel stood on one side of the table, while I stood on the other. Daniel was holding Rosa in his hands, and while we talked about Rosa and tarantulas in general, Daniel allowed Rosa to climb about his shoulders and chest. Occasionally he would stroke her furry legs as if she were a purring cat. Real cute.

While we talked, I became more and more comfortable with Rosa. When I first entered the meeting room, I was flushed and anxious. But a few simple relaxation techniques helped to alleviate this anxiety. I'm sure my therapist could see that I was becoming more comfortable with Rosa, because he asked if I minded if Rosa could walk on the table.

On the table. The table in front of me. A live tarantula. Was this a dream I was having? Could this be real? A year before, I could barely look at a picture of one, and now I was agreeing to have this spider crawl on a table directly in front of me. With absolutely no hesitation, I said, "No problem." I watched Daniel carefully remove Rosa from where she was resting at the base of his neck, and he lowered her to the table.

I watched every movement of her legs on the table as she slowly walked in front of Daniel. She was so quiet, and almost graceful in her movements, that I was totally unprepared for what happened next. All of a sudden and without warning, Rosa darted from the middle of the table and ran towards me like a gazelle from a lion. This unexpected twist in behaviour caused me to jump backwards and hold my breath. I closed my eyes and pictured Rosa flying through the air and landing on my chest. But when I opened my eyes and saw Rosa safely in Daniel's arms, I could only laugh out loud. Although Rosa had startled me, I didn't feel afraid. Any lasting anxiety I held drifted away, and I knew at that moment I no longer had arachnophobia. I had graduated and walked across the stage.

Now, when I sing "The Itsy Bitsy Spider" to my son, I always have a smile on my face. He loves it when I use my fingers to pretend a spider is crawling up his arm. A few years ago, I would have cringed at the idea of singing a song about spiders, but I no longer live in the shadow of a phobia and I no longer allow it to negatively impact my life. Like the spider in the song, it's taken determination and perseverance to overcome my uphill battle, but the end result was success. After many years of living with arachnophobia, I can now look at the beautiful and intricate spiders' webs around my home and feel satisfaction and contentment rather than anxiety and fear.

WHAT NO ONE SEES

Jill Beaton, St. John's, NL

My first few days as a patient at the Waterford Hospital were all about survival. Aside from the personal crisis that landed me there in the first place, there were a whole host of new and unpleasant things to adapt to. There was the pervasive smell of unwashed bodies. In the summer there was the unrelenting heat caused by no air conditioning and windows that don't open. The very few windows that do open are limited to two or three inches of fresh air, practically useless against the permanent stuffiness of the ward. I was mixed in with patients with all sorts of different diagnoses, some of whom were very intimidating. In my case the intimidation consisted of bullying men demanding money and cigarettes; they knew I was new and afraid, and they took advantage of it until I got my bearings and learned to stand up for myself. I also had a significant problem with sexual harassment from a couple of the male patients. For some reason there seemed to be nothing any of the staff could do about this, so I had to live with it until those men were discharged. And of course, there is the complete and total lack of privacy. For close to half of my month-long stay I shared a room with six other women. This room was completely open; there are no privacy curtains. When I asked about this I was told it was for my own protection. Much of my experience there left me feeling as if I needed to be protected from the people who were "protecting" me.

Despite the fact that this particular stay in the summer of 2006 was not my first, I was terrified. I had been there before but it can be an extremely scary place. I had to learn to survive there all over again. It had taken my psychologist, my very committed and loving psychologist, a solid month to convince me even to consider being hospitalized again. Aside from all I have just said, I think my main fear was the fear of giving up control: control over when I ate, when I slept, when I showered. Of course, my life was already very much out of control, but I was too sick to recognize it. In the days leading up to my hospitalization I worked to build up my resolve that this could help where nothing else could, and trust that this experience would not be a damaging one. Still, with every step I took, from admitting to my ward, I could feel my courage leaking away.

After the first few days I again became acclimatized to life at the Waterford and I knew I would be able to endure my time there. Things became less black and white; they had been almost exclusively black of course, with everything at first seeming unbearable. Shades of grey slowly began to enter the picture; there was a lot of bad but a little good too. There were a few staff members whom I found to be very lacking in sensitivity and empathy, although I'm sure that's true of any collection of people. But for every disagreeable person working on the unit there were at least two kind-hearted and compassionate ones. One nurse in particular was exceptionally sympathetic and generous. Nighttimes were especially hard for me, and when I was upset she would sit and talk with me for as long as I needed. One night in particular I was really in distress and she stayed and helped me work things out despite the fact that her shift had already ended.

Another problem I had was time. Time passes very slowly in that hospital; there are no set activities, and aside from mealtimes and visits from my doctors, no structure at all. The minutes dragged painfully by. But as time went on this also became less of a problem: I was allowed off the unit and discovered the cafeteria and library, and when a friend I had made on my ward was also given the privilege of going outside, it allowed us to regain some sense of normalcy in our days. It was easy to forget I was a patient in a hospital; we were just two friends having a coffee in the sunshine.

This leads me to the best, and most unexpected, part of my experience at the Waterford: the abundance of love and support I got from the other patients. Certainly, this doesn't apply to some of the patients who were there, but everyone who is there is there because they are sick and hurting. I became very close with some of the other patients, and I discovered the basic human kindness that lies within most people, even when they are going through some of the worst times in their lives. Of course it was intensely stressful living in a stuffy room with six other women, but I couldn't have asked for a better support group. They loved me, they hugged me, they gathered around me when I cried. They shared with me, their possessions but also their experiences, wisdom and strength. They greatly enhanced my hospital experience and I made some meaningful friendships that I still have to this day.

Before being admitted to hospital I was tremendously resistant to the idea. I was emphatic that I would never allow myself to be hospitalized again. But between the highly competent medical care I received and the gift of loving kindness I experienced from other patients, staying at the Waterford turned out to be one of the best things I could ever have done for myself.

YOU DON'T KNOW ME ANYMORE

Justin Ducey, St. John's, NL

I am twenty-two years old and ever since I could remember I always did badly in school. I was always fighting, disrupting class, and getting sent to the principal's office. I was tested in elementary school for ADHD (attention deficit hyperactivity disorder) but according to the results I didn't have any such thing. I was always an active kid and was told that's just the way I am. My parents tried to direct my energy towards a sport; so I got into ice hockey. I really enjoyed playing hockey but my marks didn't improve and my behaviour was still a problem in class.

When I entered junior high I was thirteen. I decided it was my last year of ice hockey. I just wanted to hang out with friends and play street hockey. This was about the time I started drinking and smoking. My marks were still suffering, my behaviour still a problem. I failed grade seven and was put in summer school.

In grade eight I was still a problem and still having problems with school work. I was taken out of some French classes and put in for extra English. I did those classes in the sped rooms (special education classes). I did manage to get through that year.

Grade nine proved that I didn't really need French — I was taken out of it completely and put in for yet more English classes. However, summer saw me returning once more to summer school. I had failed two core courses. I did one in summer school and they pushed me ahead for the other. I often got the feeling they did that so that they wouldn't have to put up with me for another year.

Then came high school and we all know what it's like — parties, new people, and I didn't care about the school aspect. I was used to getting bad grades by then. I had been smoking weed for some time now, but I would never get high during school. I was still pretty active — getting sent to the active regularly, but I didn't fight as much, possibly because of some maturity.

Maturity or not, my marks were still pretty bad. It took me five years to complete high school. The fifth year would be the turning point in my life. That year I smoked weed in school because I thought, What was the worst that can happen? Apparently, I should have said, What's the best that can happen? Because my marks shot through the roof. I remember one class in particular. The teacher took me outside at the end of class and told me that if my behaviour didn't change for the next class I wouldn't be coming back. So the next class I started to smoke weed, and at the end of class, my teacher took me out again and said, "Whatever you did this class, keep it up." So, then it started. I smoked weed for almost every class. I was doing considerably better. Instead of getting 30s, 40s, and 50s, I was getting 70s, 80s, and 90s.

I smoked weed and drank a lot. I turned nineteen throughout the year and I did a considerable amount of drinking. In fact, the previous summer there weren't ten days that I was sober. Halfway through the school year, New Year's 05-06, I went to a New Year's party. I was "getting on the load" as we called it. I was halfway through my 40-ounce bottle of Lamb's and was feeling more tired than drunk when a friend asked if I would like to try some cocaine. I said, "I am not putting nudding up my nose." So he said, "We can roll a bit up in some tobacco." Being a drunk idiot, I agreed. We smoked it. I felt brand new, not tired, or screwed up, just awake and drunk. After that point, whenever I felt tired I got him to smoke another one. That continued throughout the night and into the early hours of the morning. In fact the last one we smoked was at 11 a.m.

At that time there was a knock on the door and it was my mom. She wanted me to come home for family dinner. Like hell that was happening, because I was completely wasted. A little while later we left the party house because we were the only ones up, so we "adventured" to our other buddy's house.

That's when I passed out on my buddy's couch. Not five minutes later he started playing his electric guitar and I jumped up like a bolt of lightning and took off home. When I got home I was feeling extremely "sketched out." From that time on I had a really hard time. For two weeks I couldn't sleep and I couldn't eat. If my family cooked, I had to get away from the smell, or I felt like I would puke. I would break down and ball for no reason at all. I felt like complete garbage constantly. Eventually those feelings started to simmer down but were replaced with feelings of paranoia, and anxiety. I even thought fast food restaurants were drugging my food.

About two months later I was feeling a bit better and went to a party. I had decided to give up weed. I had a flask and a bottle of wine. I drank my flask pretty quickly but didn't get the slightest buzz. So then I decided to smoke a joint. Halfway through I had quite the buzz. I continued partying by opening my wine, but, boy, did I pay for it! The next morning I felt just like the way I did the first week I was sick. From that point I quit drinking and smoking weed. I still had some paranoia, anxiety, and now I had depression. I couldn't go out with my friends because of the temptations.

I started to go see psychiatrists. They mostly got a brief description of what happened, and a bit of family history, and then put me on some medication. I was on a couple of medications and they didn't help that much. That's when I met Dr. Walsh.

For the first little while we would talk about what was happening with me and what medication would be good for me. Eventually we found the right ones. They worked extremely well. I felt good and started to think about my future and then a little miracle happened. My aunt works on Palliative Care, and Donna Kavanagh (College of the North Atlantic–Waterford Bridge Road Centre) volunteers there.

Carolyn told her about me, and soon Mom and I had a meeting with her to discuss post-secondary.

This branch of the college works in partnership with Eastern Health. Early on when I started, Donna noticed that I had a hard time paying attention. She expected that I might have a learning disability. She got me tested. I have dyslexia — which means I have problems with reading and writing. I also found out that in some areas I am actually above average. Because of my learning disability I use special technology: Dragon and Kurzweil. Those software programs put me on an equal playing field. Now school is much easier.

I was doing well academically but still had problems with attention. Donna and I went to see Dr. Walsh to tell him she suspected I had ADHD. He agreed. He started me on medication. Within the next couple of days there was a huge change. I was actually able to focus on my work. Then we started to look at careers. I had several trades courses and decided on one. However, later, because of the technology and medication, I realized I could do more.

Currently I am doing academic math (I did general in school), physics (barely ever did that), and a post-secondary communications course to prepare me for engineering. I hope to be a geomatics engineer.

A while ago I told Donna that she didn't know me anymore. I feel I have really changed. I am more confident and I believe in myself more than I ever did.

FROM WHERE THEY ARE
TO WHERE THEY SHOULD BE

Donna Kavanagh, St. John's, NL

"I cannot describe to you the feeling of standing by and watching your friends continue to march to adulthood as you stand paralyzed. I cannot describe the pain of observing their uncomprehending faces as they struggle to understand something that even you, the person going through it, cannot. I cannot describe the pain of being forgotten and discarded by most around you. I cannot describe the pain of accepting your status as written off. I may not be able to adequately describe the pain, but I can describe the effect on one's dignity. It is destroyed. Little remains."

It is through the words of my students that I have come to understand, somewhat, the struggle of mental illness. It is through my involvement with them that I have learned the true meaning of resilience. It is through working together with the education and health care systems, and the person and family, that I have learned that there is always hope and that recovery is more than possible.

The young man whose words I have quoted above was one of many students who taught me more lessons than any professor or textbook ever could. We assisted him in getting his high school, and bridged for him to go to university. From there he won a scholarship to law school. Today he is a successful lawyer and President of the Canadian Mental Health Association, Newfoundland and Labrador Division. His work in education and advocacy is ground-breaking.

Through my journey of thirty-five years as a teacher of students with psychiatric illnesses, I have come to recognize the challenges and barriers that students overcome. I feel privileged to journey with them, from where they are, to where they should be.

Those enrolled in our centre [College of the North Atlantic's Waterford Bridge Road Centre] suffer the stigma of "high school drop out," and "mentally ill." They show their resilience by their presence. They often arrive feeling "stupid," "incapable," or as one student told me, "black." But they have still come, taking a chance that maybe this time things will be different.

If there is one commonality it is low self-esteem and confidence. Illness has often struck in adolescence — symptoms causing not only difficulty in school but in all other aspects of life. It is not just the debilitating symptoms that cause such pain but also the feeling of being different, not fitting in, being alone. Stigma, as one student told me, "wraps itself around you, choking you, making it impossible to move." The pain is real, the victims, the person and family.

A father once said to me, "It was like someone took my son and gave me back someone I did not know, someone with a lot of problems." The same man also articulated to me the stigma of mental illness when he said, "When my son had to leave school he was gone for months. No one called. I believe if my son had any other illness, even cancer, there would have been lots of calls."

While I fully recognize the barriers, it has been my experience that things can change dramatically, once the proper supports have been put in place. As one student told me recently, "You don't know me anymore." I was uncertain what he meant and asked him. He replied that he felt he had changed in many ways. This bright, articulate young man had taken five years to complete the general program in high school.

When we met he felt he was unprepared for college. He came to us to refresh his skills and look at career options. He felt he needed support if he was ever going to be successful in post-secondary. He suffered from anxiety and depression, but perhaps his biggest barrier was his low self-esteem. It was evident almost immediately that he had attention problems and that he struggled academically. Working with him we came to realize that he had an undiagnosed learning disability. Testing confirmed this, and technology and accommodations saw him progress rapidly. However, he still struggled with attention. Together he and I met with his doctor, and told him what was happening. He was treated for ADHD. Everything changed. This young man saw his potential for the first time. It was this new, confident young man he was referring to, one who could concentrate, is a math whiz, and could get 90s. In December 2009 he completed his first term in engineering with a grade point average of 3.5.

I jokingly tell my students I wish there was a confidence pill. Confidence comes from success, from getting a 90 or finishing a credit. Confidence breeds success, and we have seen much success. A young lady came to us with a diagnosis of anxiety and depression. She had been told she had a learning disability but did not know what that really meant, and how it could be accommodated. Once she learned those things she went on to complete high school, write the Florence O'Neil scholarship exam and win it. June 2008 she successfully completed a two-year college program, receiving the President's Award for Academic Excellence in the Community Support Program. She is now at university completing a degree. She is on the Dean's list. She plans to do her Master's and I know one day she'll get a Ph.D.

She's not the first to get the President's Award. Another student got one for Graphic Production. A third won it for Cooking. Several of our students have received it for Adult Basic Education. For the past five years our students have written the scholarship exam. There are five scholarships, each worth one thousand dollars. The exams are written by students in the seventeen campuses of the college [College of the North Atlantic]. Every year at least one of our students has won. Most years two did, with the exception of 2008, when three of our group got first, second and third place in the province.

Students have gone on to many different careers such as law, nursing, graphic design, graphic production, engineering, cooking, video production, visual arts, business management, machinist, community studies, and office administration.

They are now where they should be.

Donna Kavanagh is the Instructional Coordinator and also teaches in the College of the North Atlantic's Waterford Bridge Road Centre. All students in the centre have a psychiatric illness. The program is a partnership between education and health. It has been in place since September 1973. The ratio of teachers to students is one to eight. The teachers become part of the students' mental health teams. An individual plan is designed with each person to overcome barriers that have prevented them from succeeding previously. Most students complete high school at the centre, but some students attend to upgrade marks or refresh skills. The centre also assists students to bridge to post-secondary.

DISCOVER AND REDISCOVERY

Owen Bauld, Wings Point, NL

Mental illness has been a part of my life since a very early age — eight or nine, maybe ten or eleven, definitely — although at that time I wasn't aware of what the exact problems were.

And these problems — obsessive-compulsive disorder (OCD) and depression — went undetected for the better part of my life.

One of my earliest memories of being affected by mental illness was late in 1980, at age eleven. I remember sitting alone in my room in my little rocking chair, which I was extremely attached to, in the dark listening to the radio, VOCM. The only light in the room was from traffic flashing in the window and the glimmer from the light in the living room around my bedroom door. A new song, which I'd only heard a few times, came on the radio, and I remember this lonely feeling came over me, but this feeling wasn't from the way the song made me feel, it reflected how I was feeling.

The song sounded painful, aching, although I didn't know any of the words or even who was singing it; it was how I'd been feeling for some time at that particular age, but it wasn't mere loneliness or sadness I was feeling, it was something more. IT was all consuming, overwhelming and debilitating.

Sitting in my chair in my empty room, all I could do was exist in that way, in a state of misery.

This came and went but eventually stayed with me for years to come. I went to bed that night, as I always did, and said two prayers, a family prayer and the Lord's Prayer. I knelt on my bed with my hands folded on the headboard and said each prayer as fast as I could, rapidly and robotically, not even listening to the words I was saying, but it was something I simply had to do.

I now picture God above looking at me then like a cross school teacher saying, "Slow down, boy, slow down."

But this was an obsessive-compulsive act which I did from early childhood to early adulthood. When I finally stopped this behaviour, I can't recall.

Strangely though, I never thought, even in my darkest moments, that there was anything mentally wrong with me. I'd heard of depression and a little about obsessive-compulsive disorder from the media but I didn't think it applied to me.

Only in adulthood did I seriously begin to suspect there may be mental health problems, as I learned more about this subject. At age twenty, a psychiatrist diagnosed me with a chemical imbalance in my brain, which in my ignorance, I assumed showed up in a blood test, but I was wrong, as a blood test would not reveal such a thing.

For many years, I existed thinking this was my one and only problem, and I went to my doctors' appointments and took their prescribed medications blindly, asking few questions.

Finally at age thirty-five, yet another psychiatrist correctly diagnosed me with OCD and depression. At first, I thought this was only a temporary problem and that I would soon be cured of my strange and troubling thoughts and behaviour. Again, I was wrong.

OCD is a lifelong problem, and when my psychiatrist told me this, it immediately scared me. The thought of living with this mental illness for the rest of my life was daunting and worrisome.

But today with the proper medication — Olanzapine, Paroxetine and Seroquel — I have a healthier mind and a happier life and I'm better prepared than ever to live my life.

If anything positive has come from my battle with mental illness it's that I've learned to be more compassionate and understanding of other people and the ordeals they may be going through in their daily lives; as mental illness is an invisible problem, it shows in someone's eyes, but unlike a broken limb, you can't see it.

Unfortunately, the stigma, or more specifically, the abuse of the mentally ill is visible. You can see it not only in the fears of uneducated people but also in the attitude and demeanour of mental health providers: arrogant and uncaring psychiatrists and ignorant staff of mental health institutions.

Often, the mentally ill are meant to feel "wrong," as if it's their fault they're mentally ill and they've done something in their life to bring it onto themselves.

But there is absolutely nothing a mentally ill person has done to bring such an illness on, and each and every individual can be proud of who they are and their accomplishments, with a clear conscience and hold their heads high, knowing they no longer have to suffer in silence.

WHEN I FELL . . . I GOT BACK UP

Cyril S. Shugarue, Jr., St. John's, NL

Dedicated to Sean M. Sullivan, who died tragically in January 2004.

For the past quarter century of my life battling mental illness has been something that I feel is eternal; however, due to multi-pronged treatment, which for me consists of medication, a good doctor, and a loving and supportive family, it is possible to live a productive and fulfilling life.

For those of you who are reading this, allow me to elaborate that there "Was" a time in my life not so long ago when doctors, family, and myself were beginning to lose hope.

However, after two failed marriages, numerous encounters with the justice system (including being incarcerated several times) and nearly fifteen years of alcohol and drug abuse, I found my way to St. John's (and at the time homeless) where I live today, and quite happily, I might add.

Happiness for me did not come easily or magically upon moving to the city. For a brief period of time I continued to drink heavily and not listen to my doctor, or anybody else for that matter.

I was going through another separation and eventual divorce, compounded by the fact that I missed my children, then ages twelve and nine, which were from my first marriage. I was grieving badly and was certainly not looking long-term and needed immediate pain relief. That's where alcohol came into the equation for me.

Just when I thought things couldn't get any more desperate I received news that my second cousin, next door neighbour, classmate and close childhood friend had committed suicide.

At first I had no real reaction! But when it came time to go back to my hometown of Harbour Grace, where I just left, to attend a funeral . . . that was very sobering for me (literally).

This tragedy had such a deep impact on me that, even to this day, it is still very emotional for me. However, having said that, I have tried to apply something positive out of that happening when struggling with my own diagnosis of bipolar disorder.

Today I appreciate my family much more. I appreciate the strengths and talents God has given me to use to the maximum of my ability. I appreciate four and a half years of relatively stable wellness. I appreciate a great doctor/patient relationship that has been the cornerstone to my success. I appreciate life, and despite struggles that still occur and no doubt will continue to occur, I take them in stride and most importantly, "When I fall . . . I get back up!"

I would like to thank all who have read my submission and as well, for this opportunity.

EPIPHANY 6, B
Mark 1:40-45

Kate Crawford, St. John's, NL

A sermon delivered by Rev. Dr. Kate Crawford at Gower Street United Church, St. John's, February 15, 2009.

(A member of the choir stands up behind me and sounds a small "singing bowl." Its sound is clear and piercing. It hangs in the air for a moment or two.)

What you have just heard is a Tibetan Singing Bowl. It is an instrument of prayer in an ancient Buddhist culture. Buddhists "invite" the singing bowl as they begin their time of mindful meditation. It is a deeply holy sound.

(The bowl will continue to "speak" for the rest of the sermon. Those who are reading the sermon may wish to tap a filled water glass or ring a chime.)

I have asked Linda Hogan to preach with me today by sounding this singing bowl for us. It will be a holy sound for us as well, but in a slightly different way. Instead of inviting us to meditation it will be calling us to a different kind of mindfulness: all around the world, someone commits suicide every 40 seconds.[1]

A man with leprosy came to Jesus and begged him on his knees, "If you are willing, you can make me clean."

A man with leprosy came. A man with leprosy came to Jesus. Remember leprosy? The terrifying skin disease of Bible times, probably a conflation of numerous current medical conditions, everything from boils to rashes to what we now call Hansen's Disease.[2] It turned the skin on Moses' sister Miriam as white as snow

(Numbers 12:10); it turned the mighty military commander Naaman into an outcast (2 Kings 5:1); it led to the almost unbearable condition of being declared ritually unclean.

Leviticus 13:45. The person with such an infectious disease must wear torn clothes, let their hair be unkempt, cover the lower part of their face and cry out, "Unclean! Unclean!" As long as they have the infection they remain unclean. They must live alone; they must live outside the camp.

Outside the camp. A deadly prescription in a desert society. Outside the camp there were wolves. Outside the camp there was no water. Outside the camp the vultures watched wickedly, waiting to pick off the lonely, the injured and the sick.

A man with leprosy came. A man with leprosy came to Jesus. Thank God we don't have to deal with lepers anymore! The biblical bugbear has been dispelled, the bogeyman of uncleanliness is long behind us, the doors of the medieval Lazarets are closed, those pestilential warehouses for the incurably sick.

Or are they? We've still got the Waterford. Oh I know, it's not a mental hospital anymore. It's a residential care facility for people with mental illness . . . and a diabetes clinic. I think they threw in the diabetics to try to soften the image. "Yeah, sure, b'y, I'm off to the Waterford to get my dose of dialysis." Makes it sort of normal-sounding.

But for a certain generation of Newfoundlanders the Waterford was a lunatic asylum. A place to be feared. A leper colony of sorts, right on the edge of town. Outside the camp. "Mother started to get poorly after the baby died. Couldn't get out of bed, poor dear. We had to take her over to the Waterford. It was her nerves."

We may not have leprosy anymore. But we sure have lepers. "Unclean! Unclean!" as it says in Leviticus . . . for the most part we're scared to death of mental illness.

I have a friend who struggles with depression. Some terrible things happened to her in her life — I don't need to give you the details. She was doled out more pain than one person should have to live with. And although she's a survivor, although she's strong, although she put it all behind her, a dark curtain started to fall over her life. Despair. Apathy. An "eternal sadness within," to use the words of one suicide-survivor.[3]

Depression is a risk factor for developing cancer, it is a predictor of poor outcome or even death for people with cardiac disease, and raises your risk of dying after a heart attack by four times. Depression increases your risk of stroke, epilepsy, diabetes, Alzheimer's disease, cancer and even obesity. At any one point in time 4-5% of Canadians are coping with depression; 90% of them will never seek treatment.

A man with leprosy came to Jesus. And begged him on his knees. You bet he begged him. On his knees, hands pressed together in supplication, face in the dust, tears streaming down his face, a look of longing mixed with fear on his importunate face. We'd be on our knees, too, if Jesus came to town. And we had leprosy. On our knees. Looking up. Imploring that amazing man who cast out demons, who taught with authority, not as the teachers of the law used to teach.

"Please," we would say. "Please, sir," we would say. "Please take it away. Please make me clean. Please lift the darkness out of my soul. Please let me live again." Wouldn't we? I would. I would beg.

But this man, this man in Mark's gospel doesn't beg. He retains his dignity — despite the skin rotting and falling off his body, despite the scarf pulled across the lower portion of his face, as prescribed in the priestly rules of Leviticus. Despite the smell of him. He is on his knees — as before a king. But he does not beg. Listen to his words: "If you are willing, you can make me clean. If you are willing, you can make me clean."

That is not a question, is it? That is not asking for anything. "If you are willing, you can make me clean." That is a statement of fact. A simple conditional clause.[4]

It's even simpler in Greek: *Thelo*, he says. *Thelo*. One word, meaning: if you are willing.

And Jesus answers in one word: *Katharistheti*. I am willing. I am willing. The man on his knees says, *Thelo*; and Jesus responds, *Katharistheti*.

Don't you think, somehow, that the whole gospel is summed up in that one word of Jesus'? Isn't the whole point of the incarnation, God loving the world so much and giving us the only-begotten son, isn't the point of that *katharistheti*, I am willing? Isn't the whole point of Jesus' ministry, of teaching with authority, of telling stories that break open good news, of healing the blind and the sick and the lame, of sharing food with outcasts, isn't the whole point of that *katharistheti*, I am willing? Isn't the whole point of the crucifixion, the annihilation, the surrender, *katharistheti*, I am willing?

He is willing. He came. He walked among us. He didn't leave us alone. He drew close. Emmanuel. God with us. We are not alone, we live in God's world. God is here. God is always here. God has promised to be.

A man with leprosy came to Jesus and begged him on his knees. "If you are willing (*Thelo*) you can make me clean." Filled with compassion, Jesus reached out his hand the touched the man. "(*Katharistheti*) I am willing."

(*The singing bowl is silenced*). My friend found a therapist. She goes every week and talks about what happened to her. Sometimes it pours out of her in tears. Sometimes she rages and howls. But it's coming out. And it's going away. Disappearing.

Every day when she wakes up in the morning she takes a little white pill — an antidepressant. She told me it sure beats the alcohol and cigarettes she used to use to dull the pain. She takes her little white pill and goes on about her day in peace. She is a social worker. With mentally and physically disabled adults. She has become a source of safety and of healing. *Katharistheti*.

I have never coped with depression. Not yet, anyway. But if the statistics are valid, then six or seven people in this room right now have some form of it. And probably forty or so of us know someone who does. I do. I know more than one.

And I stand in awe of each one of them. Because they are so

strong. Because they are so courageous. Because they are so digni-fied. Down on the knees, yes — but as before a king. Not begging. Asking. *Thelo?* If you are willing, you can make me clean.

And we hear today — we hear it every day — but especially we hear it today. I am willing. *Katharistheti.* I am willing.

Filled with compassion, Jesus reached out his hand and touched the man . . . Be clean! Immediately the leprosy left him and he was cured.

---

1   Facts on suicide and depression are taken from *Quick Facts: Mental Illness and Addiction in Canada.* The Mood Disorders Society of Canada, 2006.

2   See James Orr, "Leper; Leprosy" in *The International Standard Bible Encyclopedia*: http://www.studylight.org/enc/isb/view.cgi?number=T5483

3   from "Nancy's Story," in *Changing Minds*, CMHA-NL video clip: http://www.cmhanl.ca/minds.asp#cmclips

4   The development of this idea and what follows is based on Scott Hoezee, "Questions to Ponder/Issues to Address" at The Center for Excellence in Preaching: http://cep.calvinseminary.edu/thisWeek/index.php

DESPERATE DESIGN

Amanda Penney, Mount Pearl, NL

I was in the hospital, convinced that I was pregnant. I would not take my medication because I thought that it would harm the baby. Finally, I agreed to take the pills. They had a very strong effect on me. It was like I was asleep and awake at the same time. I thought that I was going into labour. I felt and heard them wheel me out of the bedroom into the delivery room. I spread my legs and remember a woman saying, "She's helping us." So then I pushed and wet my bed, thinking that I had just given birth to twins, yet in reality I was just lying in a bed coated with my own urine. I thought that my twins were born missing body parts and said, "Take anything you need to help them." The next day I thought that I had no skin even though the mirror clearly showed otherwise. I actually felt a line of pain going down my stomach, thinking that they had taken out a few organs to help the twins by cutting me open the night before, and that they had used some new technology to fix the surgery cuts so that you could not see them at all. I thought that my deformed twins were sold by the doctors. This was one of my more recent episodes.

It all started when I was thirteen. The changes in my personality were staggering . . . I went from an outgoing, confident, charismatic girl to an isolated, quiet, self-absorbed mess with no self-esteem. I would escape by sleeping and spending my waking hours as a character in a video game. I would get in vicious fights with my mother.

I would miss school. I stopped calling my friends. After awhile my friends gave up on me. I had given up on life.

One night Mom and I got into a massive fight. When she was upstairs I took a knife out of the kitchen drawer and sat on the floor rocking back and forth repeating two words, "I hate." Then I cut my wrist in three spots. When I think back it was more of a cry for help than a suicide attempt. The ambulance took me to the Janeway psychiatric ward. I did not like talking to doctors. Often I would stare at them with eyes full of anger and not respond to their many questions. I would then go into my room and listen to "Runaway Train" and "#1 Crush" and cry.

I did not like the hospital with its many rules and needles. Some aspects of being in the hospital left bigger imprints on me. I had broken one of the rules. A nurse came over and told me to get off the phone. I would not. Finally I was pulled away and the receiver broke because I would not let go. I was crying and yelling so they put me in the "Quiet Room." I pounded my head, fists and elbows on the door, screaming for them to let me out. "Not until you calm down!" They never realized that as long as I was in that small room I could not be calm. By the time a doctor came in to give me a needle to stop my hysterical behaviour, my arms looked mutilated because they were so swollen and bruised.

Once a doctor gave me a rubber band to put on my wrist, and said that whenever I have a negative thought to snap it. When she came back my wrist was raw from all of my bad thoughts.

Fast Forward — I was in the Janeway again because of an overdose. As soon as I turned sixteen they released me immediately. They had been subjected to enough of my attitude, I'm sure. I was taking my medication for my depression which seemed to be working. Though I always felt tired. I pitied myself because I had lost all of my friends. I quit school in grade eight. I tried going to different schools to no avail. I found it was too stressful and I worried so much about what other people thought of me. I often found expressing myself through my artwork would bring me solace. I have always had talent when it came to drawing pictures.

Years later I was twenty-one and doing great. Working at Wal-Mart and going downtown on the weekend with my friends. I started going out with this charmer who had just moved to Newfoundland from Africa. After around a year we moved away to Winnipeg. For awhile things were great. I was working full-time telemarketing and was often the top seller for weeks in a row and was living with who I thought was the love of my life . . . Well he cheated and a lot of bad stuff happened.

I got on a plane and went home. I had to go into the Waterford Hospital because I was having my first manic episode and it was a doozy. They kept trying me on different medications with no success. I gained forty pounds in less than two months from side effects of the medications. Then it was decided that I would have shock therapy. It made me forget so much of my past. I remember my mom telling me that "Some things are best off forgotten." I was diagnosed with borderline personality disorder and bipolar.

Mania would rear its head in very embarrassing forms. When I am manic I never realize until it is too late. I would hear a song on the radio and get angry, thinking that they stole my lyrics. I would think that certain television shows were made just for me to tell me secrets. I would dance like crazy in front of everyone in the smoke room. I would become very aggressive verbally with certain people. At times I felt like my brain was on fire. I thought that this was caused when I had an EEG done. I thought that they put wires inside my head through the coloured holes in the cap. I was even contemplating shaving my head to show the nurses that there were wires implanted in my brain. I would get into the bath or shower with my clothes on then walk down the hall naked. I would then say I was naked because . . . "my clothes were wet." I was often suicidal.

The last time I tried to kill myself was years ago. It was my most serious attempt. I filled up the bathtub and got in with my pyjamas on. I had the hair dryer in one hand and the toaster in the other. I dropped them both in. I kept getting shocks all through my body yet

I was still very much alive. I stumbled and twitched my way out of the bathtub. The toaster still worked! I never told anyone that I did that.

A few people called me a "retard" when they heard that I was in the Waterford Hospital. I was so ashamed. I tried to hide and deny that I had an illness. I would stop taking my pills, stop going to the doctor, and over time I would get more and more sick. I was drinking heavily and smoking a lot of weed among other things. I would steal liquor from my mom and get drunk by myself. I felt worthless.

Buzz
The sugar is all gone.
The red-eyed fiend searches the cracks in the floor picking up each crystal with bristly
arms. With a flutter of fury surroundings are abandoned.
Many eyes flicker back and forth.
Appetite satiated for the moment . . . a moment is never enough.
A buzz of excitement. Bouncing against the glass.
Not even bearing the strength to crack. Already broken. Cold, always cold.
Not even noticing that the place you call home has begun to grow mould.
So young, feeling so old. Living a filthy excuse for a life. Never told.
Scraping your wealth together with a knife. Time always goes far too slow.
Not only the wind does blow. Seeking out others to fly in circles with. Never realizing that time is a gift.

My case manager told me about a government-formed program that she thought would pry me out of the downward spiral I was in. I started working at the Harbour Side Studio, getting paid to draw and paint all day. This was my dream job. I did not want to miss one day. I was losing more control of my thoughts and actions as each day went by. One morning Mom refused to drive me to work because, unlike me, she could see that I was in no state to go. I was determined and decided I would walk there. I was walking and I spied a box full of metal curtain rods and decided to take one. This would be my walking stick. I was walking along the highway and suddenly I saw that the police were blocking off traffic on both sides. What did they want with me? Were they going to take me away? I had no idea what was going on. My mom had called the police. Three policemen were walking towards me slowly. I felt threatened. I started spinning my walking stick, which was now transformed into my weapon. I held up my metal rod as if it was a baseball bat, telling them to stay away from me. This caused them to rush towards me. I swung and hit the policeman on the right in the shoulder. They quickly overpowered me and put me into cuffs. I started screaming for my dad, over and over, to help me. He could not. He had been electrocuted at work when I was six. The policeman in the car with my mom started to cry when she told them that I was calling out for a dead man.

I have overcome my need for drugs and alcohol. Now I am in control. I have to take medication every night and see my doctor monthly. I have finally accepted that these are things that I need to do to *stay* in control. I had to stop hanging around with my old circle of friends. My main support comes from my mom, Madonna, who never gave up on me.

I am now going to school at the College of the North Atlantic campus on Waterford Bridge Road to finish my high school. That is something that I thought I would never be able to do. The teachers are one of the main reasons that I am succeeding. Another is the students who do not define who I am by my illness, and who have gone through many of the same pitfalls as me — mainly the stigma that wraps itself around people who have mental illnesses. I actually have hopes and plans for the future now. I have shown my artwork at two shows and sold a good number of my drawings. My self-esteem soared when my picture *Connections* was shown in two newspapers and sold for six hundred and fifty dollars.

I have worked at Masonic Park, a home for seniors. I was helping with the art program there and working with this lady who was an accomplished artist. Since she had her stroke she could only paint half of the picture in her mind. It was up to me to help her finish the other half. I hope to eventually become an art therapist and work with patients in the various psychiatric wards and old age homes. I just need to devote myself and stay true to the fact that though sometimes it seems that every day is a struggle, I am a very strong person and that life is and always will be worth living.

That is an understatement.

POLICE OFFICER CONTRIBUTIONS TO THE IMPROVEMENT OF MENTAL HEALTH SERVICES IN NEWFOUNDLAND AND LABRADOR

Sharon Barter Trenholm, St. John's, NL

For sixteen years I have worked alongside and assisted police officers in this province as they have worked to initiate and facilitate improvements in multiple areas. One of the areas which has received a great deal of their efforts is that of responding to individuals experiencing mental health issues. The police officers of this province have played a large role in the improvement of the provision of mental health services in Newfoundland and Labrador. As a manager with the Royal Newfoundland Constabulary, I have seen the impacts on police officers who have to respond daily to calls involving mental health issues. Some of these calls end with good resolutions, some with what passes for all that can be done, and others have tragic outcomes. All police officers are impacted by what they cannot do to help. This motivates many of them to participate in seeking better ways to respond.

In 2004 the Psychiatric Assessment/Short Stay Unit opened at the Waterford Hospital. This was a key moment in policing in the province. Several dedicated police officers, RNC and RCMP, have served for years on stakeholder committees which contributed to the initiation of this unit. These are officers who for years of their careers had no choice but to convey individuals in mental health crisis to the lock-up. These officers knew this was wrong and worked for years with their partners in the health care and correctional systems to make these much-needed changes. Many of these same officers also worked to ensure the revised *Mental Health Care and Treatment Act* would meet the needs of the people of this province.

Also in 2004, the RNC began training their recruits through the new Police Studies Diploma Program at Memorial University. To be eligible to begin the program, applicants must be a graduate of a degree program or have completed university level courses in English, psychology, and sociology. Once admitted to the program they must complete courses in political science, psychology, social work, sociology, and police studies. Additionally, the third semester of practical training at the RNC Training Section includes the Changing Minds mental illness education program and informa- tion sessions on the *Mental Health Care and Treatment Act*, Mental Health Court and other related topics. By the end of their year of training the recruits are well prepared for their duties, including their anticipated assistance with responses to individuals in mental health crisis. The need for education in the increasingly complex world of policing was identified by the dedicated staff of the RNC and they worked for years with the provincial government and Memorial University to make this program a reality. There is no other program like this in the country. In a recent report on mental health training for police officers, commissioned by the Canadian Association of Chiefs of Police, the RNC recruit training was recog- nized as a national best practice.

In 2005 the Police/Mental Health Liaison Committee presented to The Standing Senate Committee on Social Issues, Science and Technology in response to *Mental Health, Mental Illness and Addiction: Issues and Options for Canada.* A member of the RNC was part of the presenting group and is also a founding member of the committee. The PMHL is sponsored by the Canadian Association of Chiefs of Police.

In 2008 the first Assertive Community Treatment Team was initiated. Initial input and continuing support from police officers will certainly help this initiative to reach its goal of providing higher levels of treatment in the community. Expansion of this program across the province will be welcomed by police officers in all communities.

Also in 2008, we saw the initiation of the Mental Health Crisis Centre, a 24-hour, seven days a week telephone and in-person crisis intervention service provided by Eastern Health. The RNC and RCMP were consulted, and assisted with the design of this service, and provide support as required so as to ensure mental health professionals can respond and be supported 24-7. This is another in a long line of daily assistance provided. This support, referrals to the Mental Health Court, and requests for community services provision are the types of things which do not make big impressions on the general public, but they positively impact those directly involved.

The reader may wonder why this list of initiatives is included amongst the essays of personal experiences. The answer is that the story of the changes needs to be told and the police officers involved will probably not tell the stories themselves as they see their efforts as part of their job, not something for which they should receive personal credit. For years police officers in this province have been working tirelessly to change the way they respond to individuals in mental health crisis situations. Because of the nature of their work, police officers do not often have cause to celebrate advancements. The work is difficult and challenging, thus it is important to pause and reflect upon positive changes which can provide the positive reinforcement to continue the quest for change.

Much of the progress seen in recent years has been due in part to the dedicated police officers of this province who have identified where change is needed and have worked with their colleagues in partner agencies and the community to bring about that change. Usually we do not see that side of the officers publicly. We often see portrayed in the media what they cannot do to help. This is a good opportunity to list some of the initiatives where police officers have helped to make a difference. I am proud of my colleagues and their dedication to their communities. Please, join me in encouraging them to keep up their efforts to continue to improve our province and the mental health services provided.

SlightDepressShun: a literary bebop jazz improvisation for Boyd Thistle

Bradley Clissold, St. John's, NL

The following piece was inspired by and is dedicated to little-known Newfoundland artist-author Boyd Thistle who currently lives and works just outside of St. John's. A lifelong sufferer of male depression, Boyd has talked with me extensively about his battles with the disease, everything from moods and medications to misdiagnoses and media misrepresentations. These imagined scenes and ideas about depression became the source materials for this creative project: an attempt to recreate through language the fluid "riffing" movements of a jazz song on the topic of male depression.

My decision to use a stream-of-consciousness aesthetic form to present a host of interpenetrating and often ironic (even contradictory) images about depression arose out of a comment Boyd once made about his disease; he said that living with depression was like playing an improvisational jazz solo, but always with a recognizable jazz standard on the theme of sadness dominating the audible background and colouring all aspects of the solo's performance.

The formal choice of a jazz aesthetic also conveniently allows this piece of writing to mimic human thought processes through witty word play and jarring image juxtapositions, akin to the abrupt cognitive shifts Boyd describes as part of his daily struggle. Designed as a piece of fiction to foreground the specific stigmas associated with male depression, the play on words in the title Slight Depress Shun (Slight Depression) foregrounds, from the outset, that the subject of this piece is the dismissive social and cultural attitudes (slight and shun) that surround frank discussions about male depression.

SlightDepressShun. Who? Me? You? Too? Them? Us. *We are the world.* Trapped in our cells, our selves. Cell mates. Mating cells. Metastasization. House arrested on corruption charges. *From the bottom to the top, the top to the bottom.* Burning the candle at both ends just to make ends meet. Happy pills for sad days: happy daze are here again. *Nothin' to do, no where to go-oh. I want to be sedated.* Just a little something to help take the edge off of the precipice that you continue to dance along with incomplete abandon. I am man, hear me whimper into a feigned public cough, while I whisper to a scream in the places where blind newts, who will never see the light of day, savour the flavour of rotting and decomposing resentment. They won't scatter, and they don't scurry at the approach of lost tourists flip-flopping along with flashbulbs lighting their path. Silenced into self, secluded suicide watched, *till* stammering *human voices wake us and we drown,* into civil warring wondering what recent resent meant: *What we've got here is failure to communicate.* Resent from where? Resent from whom? From this living dead letter office? What is the status of the compartment where they store all undelivered missives gone astray to be redirected and bound to be resent?: full. Backing down one-way streets; backing up beyond and past the past like a drunk-driving angel of history steering using the rear-view mirror. *And if you love him, be proud of him, after all he's just a man. Stand by your* meds. Bouncing along rock bottom like an unthinking cod, the water carrier carrying water carried deep in waterlogged carriages is bursting at the seems to be. Speak your mind, just mind the gap. Which way to reality? How far? Are we there yet? Are there any shortcuts? Is there anything a little nicer? Maybe a little closer? With a better view? Can we change the colours? Around the same price range, perhaps? Do you mind taking a picture of us (as we want to remember today and be remembered tomorrow)? Framed and convicted. *La réalité est une illusion créée par l'absence de drogue.* Distorted unhealthy ways of thinking. Cellular shrinking. Neuronal death. A hurt sense of reality. One flew under the radar and over the cuckoo's nest. Withdraw. Withdrawn. Without. Area 25 of the brain. Standard deviations. Drug it down, talk it down, shock it down, to feel up. Change is the symptom, the cause, and the cure. Push away, pull back, runaway, but it runs too deep in the family. Inherit the sad. Better-off-without-me thoughts. Before my mother wore glasses, she didn't know there were individual leaves on tall trees. *I beg your pardon. I never promised you a rose garden. Along with the sunshine, there's gotta be a little rain sometime.* Black minutes blackened by the bluest blues. SlightDepressShun it's just electro shock away; SlightDepressShun *it's justa kiss away, kissaway, kissaway, kiss away.* Flash flood! Tread water softly staying afloat atop the gaping depths that you have charted where fish glow neon with malicious intent, where the sun cannot shine, where nothing grows that does not prey upon or get preyed upon. Truly gone fishing. Take a cannibalistic Time-Out to self-masticate the inside of your cheek, lost in thought, oblivious to the passerby world: keep on gnawing.

Get to the wicket, buy you a ticket. Go. Go.

In meds we trust. Haha, haha.

All you need are meds. Boppopopopah.

I'm a broken man on a Newfoundland *pier.*

What's appear?

A disappointed bridge.

To nowhere fast. Standing at the edge of the sea, at the end of the continent. Inconsolable. Incognito. Incontinent. Incongruity. *I see a world that's tired and scared of livin' on the edge too long, where does she get off tellin' me that love could save us all.* You say friends and I only hear the last four letters. You use the C-word commitment. And I think of the committed masses who watch ultra-blue late-night televisual flickerings in lonely bedroom windows. Married rhymes with buried, always has and always will, and settling down is a downward settling of affairs. *Letting the days go by. Let the water hold me down. Letting the days go by. There is water underground. Into the blues again. Into the silenced water.* Sociopathic empathy. Misanthrope without hope. Slippery slope, rope-a-dope. Beyond the scope of nope, mope, cope. *The only thing I learned from love, was how to aim at someone who outdrew ya.* Lonely stagnant waters are breeding grounds for divorces from reality. Muddied waters look deceptively deep. You'll break your neck if you dive head first. *Look before you leap has never been the way we keep.* In a millisecond rock bottom races up to meet the free-falling breakaway elevator. Punch desperately at the buttons as you plummet: punch floors, punch alarms, punch stop. And yet rock bottom will feel like an eternity of loss and lack of control. An endless spiral staircase going down and down. Without a sound. Happiness hurts and love lashes; concern criticizes and affection afflicts with suspicion of affectation. This fall silently eats feet-per-second to get ahead of you always mindful of your mind's fullness. But by now, you don't care how the bottom ends as it meteorically rises to meet your crashing soul. Morbid thoughts paint sordid pictures of possible easy outs, but each requires too much of your apathetic agency to reach a final stop and pop your drop. Thirty thousand suicides a year. Yet she insists incessantly that there is a big difference between wanting to kill yourself and not wanting to live anymore. *And the band played Eve of Destruction.* To err is human, to forget divine, and to worry anxiously and uncontrollably about what has already happened gets packaged as internalized defeat. She's got a hurt sense of self, bruises on her soul, but you'd never know it. For her, no tuna casseroles or florist's flowers get sent to get well soon. Just get over your depression, just pick yourself up, dust yourself off, and get on with it. Why so angry? Why can't you make decisions? Thoughts of graveside services and suicide scenarios, self-defeating cancerous attitudes: harm self, harm others. *Day destroys the night and night divides the day. Try to run, try to hide, break on through to the other side.* What is the other side of black and blue? *What is the colour when black is burned? Deep* bruising that never rises to the skin's surface, but instead pains to the slightest pressure. Own it! The sun unable to penetrate the clouds that race across the sky beneath your bent head. Own it! And there are no scars to show off and prove that you're battle-proven and — weary. Own it! You continue to dance along the precipice of reason, partnered with spectres of Jacques Derrida, who line up waiting their turn to cut in when the morbid musical notes of nihilism pause. Stole it! Your dance card is full and the pained Piper knows many tunes, most of them dirges. Own it! Listen he's playing your song again. *This ain't no party! This ain't no disco! This ain't no foolin' around!* This ain't no wonderland either, Alice! And this sure ain't Kansas, Dorothy! Stick a needle in my—

Eye of the storm and nothing else matters;

and sometimes not even that.

Sometimes I just feel too much, when I don't want to feel at all.

Why can't you just wake up and get over your cancer!

How can you know the dancer from the dance? The teller from the trance? The cancer from the can'ts? Shake it off! Jus' git up, an' git on with it!

When I say hit it — hit it! And when I say quit it — quit it!

Now hit it!

Hit it!

Okay now quit it!

Quit it!

Can't play you no blues. Never had the blues, only shades of black.

No whiter shades of pale. The daze within the days; the haze within the maze; got a minotaur on my back; the too-close-to-the-sun heat melts the cracks in the wax filling my ears and securing my wings. Full fathom five freefall I fly and metaphorically lie. Slight depression is a small dent in the head: the running joke of having been dropped as a baby. How do you text message the stigma of male depression? Muddle through. Doesn't everybody find their way? Eventually? Premature ghostmodern postmortem: I brood, therefore, I am. But this is no pose, captured and froze, no Kodak moment; no immortalized and perfected BIG screen performance (multi-taken). I know no Byronic heroes who walk miserably romantic, tormented, and sexy tragic, in my neighbourhood; just keep pretending *it's a beautiful day in the neighbourhood — would you be? could you be? my neighbour?* Good fencing makes good neighbours — *en garde!* Going, going, gone underground — into hiding, man — into group therapy coupled with a strict regimen of medicated happiness and a solid twelve-hours-a-night of sedated mayhem where anxiety nightmares strike aching terror into splayed and butterflied souls; none of which they will remember in the mourning save the sharp pain at the back of their mouths where they've cracked their teeth, crown to root. *And you must make a friend of* Depression. Depression *and mortal terror are your friends; if they are not, then they are enemies to be feared.* The camera never blinks — it blacks out, then passes out on the editing-room floor — most of what you see in a film is the invisible black space between frames that shutter subliminal. I'm a stranger killing a stranger who won't surrender to a mediated reality. You end up looking down so much until you can't look up again, only go lower; downward-facing dog; you can always look down on your feet. *Born under a bad sign, been down since I began to crawl; if it wasn't for bad luck, wouldn't have no luck at all.* All is fine, but you feel no brightness, taste no sunshine; see through the world darkly that the bleak shall inherit the earth as ashed ashes and dusted dust. Men don't cry, and, when they do, nobody wants to know. *I first met Dean not long after my wife and I split up. I had just gotten over a serious illness that I won't bother to talk about, except that it had something to do with the miserably weary split-up and my feeling that everything was dead.* An unconscious and uncultivated loner *chic.* Don't show, don't tell a tale of woe or risk recrimination. The only true measure of life and love is loss: *when you ain't got nothin', you ain't got nothin' to lose.* The Chinese water torture of breathing without conviction. Pull the heavy water past your body, black and viscous with desperate memories. Out of my head, out of my mind, off my rocker, out to lunch, not quite right: SlightConfessShun; SlightDepressShun. *The Great* Id *has spoken! Pay no attention to the man behind the curtain!* Speaking in Pop-Culture Tongues — voice ventriloquy — to break bionic through the ironic moody poses of our stylized celebrity brooders paid to pout like poets. Even the economy gets depressed sometimes. *Choose the highest bidder was my answer when they told me I was up for sale.* Going out of business. Total clearance — everything must go. No refunds and no returns. All sales final. One size fits small. *These clothes don't fit us right. Time to make a change. It's all the same, it's all the same.* The only person who really knew me was my tailor because he regularly re-measured. Her golf ball found the slight depression in the ground. You keep telling me I should do my taxes: why?

Okay, one more time let's hit it!

Hit it!

And one last time let's quit it!

Quit it!

(and try to smile for them as you do it).

No sun again today. Depress the snooze button on *bursting, radiant life* a little longer.

A LIFE REVEALED

Ann Galway, Paradise, NL

I read an article a short time ago in which a woman stated that if she knew her child's teacher suffered from depression, she would pull her child from that teacher's class. I have taught school for more than thirty years and struggled with depression for longer than that. It was because of this attitude and the stigma attached to mental illness that I hid my condition from friends, colleagues, and family. I carried the shame like a burning flame inside me and it hurt me more than the depression itself. My children knew there were times when I was ill but it has only been in the past couple of years that I was able to let go of the shame long enough to talk to them about it.

I have looked back over the years and know with certainty that my first encounter with depression was while I was in my teens. I grew up in a small community at a time when Oprah and Dr. Phil would have been considered taboo. The only hint of mental illness came when someone had to be "taken away," usually during the night, and they would return months later only to have the process repeated a year or so later. Hushed whispers with words like "poor thing!" and "what a shame!" didn't encourage me to talk about how I was feeling. I learned early to put on a happy façade when around friends. Even my closest girlfriend was totally unaware.

I moved away at sixteen to go to university. I pasted a smile on my face and for the most part I fooled everyone. Girls who roomed with me heard me cry at night and asked, "What's wrong?" I never told them. Sometimes I was moody and unfriendly as I struggled to keep afloat. I got a reputation for sleeping a lot. I didn't know I was doing that to escape. To sleep was such a relief. But sometimes I was fun-loving and friendly and I caught glimpses of the person I really was. I liked that person but she never stayed for long.

I dated but I never allowed myself to get close enough for someone to learn my secret. Yes, it was beginning to feel like I was carrying around a secret and it was becoming a larger burden each day. Then I met my husband of thirty-two years now. How he was able to get me to open up and how he stood by and guided me and continued to love me is a story for another time. Let's just say, I finally started to look for help. One doctor told me all I needed was a week in Florida. I believed him. We went to Florida. A few weeks after, I found a new doctor.

After we were married I had a series of miscarriages and finally had to admit I would never carry a child. The depression hit hard and my husband insisted I seek help in St. John's. I finally got to see a real psychiatrist. The man was old, had an office in a dreary dark house on LeMarchant Road and nodded off during the session. I never went back. I was never hospitalized but a few nights after that encounter, I had to be taken to St. Clare's where I begged for help. I was told there was no bed available but I was introduced to Valium. For the next few years I couldn't leave the house without them. I also learned that alcohol could take me to brighter places where I could laugh, dance and enjoy myself. I began to look forward to the weekends.

When I came crashing down, I got myself back to St. John's and this time I was luckier. I was referred to a new psychiatrist whose office was in a similar dark, old house converted into an office. He was kind and listened. He also prescribed an antidepressant. But there was no explanation forthcoming of why this was happening to me. The shame of having to take those pills was so great that many times I stopped taking them only to have to start over again.

Every day I fought this demon. Many wonderful things happened along the way. One was the adoption of our two beautiful babies. When I felt like I was going to fall into the deep black abyss, they were the faces I focused on. My husband continued to be my biggest support. I met a wonderful doctor in one community we lived in, who was a guardian angel. There were times I had gone for several nights without sleep. This doctor came to our home to give me a sedative and was there in the morning to check on me.

I was forced to take sick leave from time to time for short periods. Quitting was not an option for me. I was determined not to give into this thing that had haunted me for so long. I fought back and I continued to work. Being in the classroom was therapeutic. I loved to teach and I loved children. Children love you unconditionally and it was a place where I didn't have to pretend. Honesty prevailed in the classroom. Adrenaline pumped through me and I gave it my all every day. It was where I felt whole and fulfilled.

We moved to a larger centre in 1993 where I found a young doctor who was to open up my world. She referred me to a psychiatrist who took the time to explain "chemical imbalance" and prescribe proper medication. His office is not hid away in some old house on a side street but is bright and welcoming. I don't hide my head in shame when I go to see him and I always leave smiling. Slowly he is teaching me to believe in myself, that I am not a "bad" person because I need a pill to keep a chemical in balance in my brain. The shame is dissipating and I am talking to my family and friends about my illness. It is a difficult process though, and I still get comments like, "But you have no reason to be depressed." I do have reason to be depressed — I have a chemical imbalance and sometimes I run out of my reserves of this chemical and need medication and counselling. This is how I see it and it works for me. I continue to have bouts of depression and at those times I rely on my past record of survival to get me through.

Now that I am retired from teaching I work harder at keeping myself busy and my mind occupied. Having retired from the province in 2001, and giving myself a year to regroup, I took a teaching position in the Northwest Territories. I worked for four more years. I take computer and writing classes and want to do photography as well. I spend as much time as I can with my two-year-old granddaughter, who has brought me new life. I am proud of my accomplishments and consider myself a survivor in every sense of the word.

I have to have faith that the medical system in Newfoundland and Labrador is going to continue to make the appropriate improvements in caring for the mentally ill. They need to make it a priority. Equally important is the growing awareness and knowledge being put out there about mental illness. It is only when the cloak of shame is lifted that people living with a mental illness like depression will be able to hold their heads high and feel free to talk to the people in their lives without fear or judgment.

THE TURMOIL INSIDE HER

Alicia Cox, Conception Bay South, NL

When I was a young girl, I never knew what mental illness really was. Although mental illness affected many people in my family, I never understood the impact it had on my life until I was much older.

My grandmother suffered from manic depression bipolar disorder all of her life. This illness is caused by a chemical imbalance in the brain. It is not a choice in lifestyle and it is not an illness that is easily controlled. My grandmother endured a life that many would never wish upon their worst enemy. She was surrounded by a very loving and supportive family, yet no love and care we gave her could help manage the turmoil inside her.

I remember being a small child when Nan, as I called her, would have one of her manic episodes. I would watch as Nan walked aimlessly around our neighbourhood from door to door, looking to talk to someone; she was talkative when in a manic state. I would wake in the night to Nan baking bread at three in the morning. We never needed the bread, but she had to find something to do with her excess energy. I never understood what was happening and all I was told was that Nan was "sick." But I knew it was not with a common cold or any physical ailment. I knew something was affecting her mind and her spirit but I did not know what it was.

At other times Nan would be so quiet and depressed that we

could not rouse her from bed. We could not get her to go out, even to dress herself some days. Before proper medication was administered she was so heavily medicated it put her into a zombie-like state for days. It was a constant up and down roller-coaster of emotions and frustration for the family, yet none of us could imagine what she was going through. Nan would move aimlessly from one extreme to the other regarding her moods and her energy levels. We all felt helpless.

My grandmother was not properly diagnosed with manic depression until 1981, but she had been ill since 1959. This means she had a twenty-two year battle with her illness before it was recognized. Until 1983 she was treated as a guinea pig for various medications and experiments, including shock therapy and isolation. I listened in horror as my mother recalled the many trips they made to the Waterford Hospital for Nan's "treatment." Yet nothing seemed to work for her. Now I realize that the disorder was not understood well enough to give proper treatment.

As I grew older and the disorder was explained to me, I finally began to piece together the memories of my childhood. It was so hard for me to explain to friends why my nan could be happy one minute and so sad the next. When they visited me for play dates I knew they wondered what was wrong, yet very few ever asked me. Of course there was such a stigma attached to mental illness that it was rarely discussed in any home back then, which made it even more difficult.

Now I realize that the stigma still exists even today. In a world with all its technology, modern medicine, space exploration and economic privilege, it seems so sad that people who have mental illness are still outcasts. They are cast aside, isolated and often ridiculed for something they have no control over. It seems bigotry, ignorance and prejudice are still all too common in society.

Again I remember when my nan would go out in the neighbourhood and we would receive phone calls from people stating, "Mrs. T is down the road again acting up. Someone better come get her." I hope to think it was not due to blatant ignorance, but rather a lack of understanding. People outside our family did not live with the situation so it was unfamiliar to them. I did not hate the people in my neighbourhood for this, but I was angry. All I wanted was for others to see my grandmother for who she really was, and not for her illness. My grandmother was a human being, not a label.

Despite the hardships she faced, Nan endured. When she began a regimented medication program and proper treatment follow-up she finally gained control of the illness that had plagued her for so long. Unfortunately, once she conquered one illness, another befell her. She lost her long battle with cancer in 2003.

My grandmother gave birth to sixteen children in all, twelve of whom survived to adulthood. From those twelve children she received many blessings in the form of grandchildren and great-grandchildren. She gave them all the best love and compassion she could render. Our family never went without anything and we always knew how much she loved us and how proud she was of all of us. She never relapsed into darkness even after tragically losing two sons later in life.

So I write this essay in memory and honour of her. She was a woman to be admired and to be remembered. Although manic depression was a part of her life, it did not consume her life. She lived every day to the fullest and never took life for granted.

I only hope that the many lessons she taught me will stay with me for the rest of my life.

My only wish is that the stigma attached to mental illness will one day be abolished and that a greater understanding and compassion will be expressed toward those that suffer from it.

WHAT? ME DEPRESSED?

Terry Rielly, Paradise, NL

When my family doctor first suggested I showed signs of having "clinical depression" I recall being, at the very least, slightly surprised. Perhaps "shocked!" is more the word.

"What? Me depressed?" I responded. Then went on to add something like, "But I make my living hanging out with teddy bears, making children and their families happy . . . I have a great life! How can I be depressed?"

Prior to that appointment it had taken a long time to accept and face up to the fact that something was very wrong in my life and there was little enthusiasm for anything except perhaps staying in bed most of the day.

Remarkably, I was able to lift myself out of the dark frame of mind and put on a fun performance for my audiences. Smiling children's faces were one thing that seemed to have the ability to at least temporarily make me feel good. Not much else could. That became more and more obvious.

My usual state of mind was gradually becoming darker and darker. Increasingly I was becoming less the sort of person people wanted to be around (or) that's how it felt. I recall wondering, "What's their problem?"

Was I suicidal? I tell (or perhaps fool) myself that I never got quite that low. Admittedly, all sorts of ways were imagined how life might end. A re-occurring one was taking a curve in the road a little too fast and plunging down a cliff. At these times, second thought always gave me some sort of excuse to nix the idea. "What if I just beat up the car?" and "What if I 'fail'? How embarrassing that would be!"

It was one afternoon when my then partner had come home that the realization hit me in the face. "No, I'm not all right." It took a bit of nerve to admit it. Sure glad I did.

As we often did, we'd check in with each other and ask what sort of day we'd had. Usually my response was, "Oh, you know — not too bad. Kind of quiet." In fact, the tendency had become to spend more and more of the day in bed. Avoiding life! When asked if I was all right that particular day, what happened next was proof enough that I was far from being well.

It was as if a long dark tunnel appeared between us, and either she was being sucked down one end of it, or I was being sucked down the other. If it had been the sixties I might have thought I was having a drug-related flashback. But it was the nineties and something was obviously terribly wrong.

Very frightened, I then added, "No, I need to see my doctor."

In fairly short order, a diagnosis of "clinical depression" was made and then confirmed when I was referred to psychologist Dr. Malcolm Simpson. Over a series of appointments, and in a relatively short period of time, Malcolm helped me realize the complexities of what I was experiencing, some of the why, and what I might consider as possible actions to take.

The road to recovery has felt long, sometimes very arduous, and really full recovery seems only like a distant possibility — at least without medication. Dark times still occur. Thank God for Mary Watson, my family doctor, for Malcolm, and yes, even the prescription drugs.

A question popped up that likely many people consider. It also occurred to me. "Should I worry about the stigma?"

And yes, I considered the larger question. Why should *anyone* have to put up with that often attached stigma while facing a struggle with mental illness? How it affects their acceptance or non-acceptance in society as a whole? Some people likely add to their illness simply trying to hide it.

Obviously I can only address how I, as an individual, respond to this common dilemma. My own "clinical depression" (and I do "own" it) is a very mild form of mental illness compared to what many others face daily.

Something else said to my family doctor as she wrote out the initial referral was, "I'm going to use this!" She gave me a rather puzzled look.

Early on in my diagnosis was the decision to learn more about mental health and the different forms it takes. Why society still (by and large) ignores that this is just one more piece in the fabric that makes up our community. In fact, I might go so far as to suggest for those who don't have a mental illness, it's an opportunity to test your own compassion, how deep your desire is for understanding, and how willing you are to accept we are all individuals and all deserve to be treated gently, kindly, and lovingly in all of our relations.

If only! Mental illness is part of life. A part of the world we live in. So, get over it, folks.

I believe statistics suggest one in five have a mental illness of some sort. With the fear of stigma attached, my guess is that survey respondents were not always completely open and honest. Like myself, not always honest with themselves either.

I am pleased to have close friendships with a couple of people who have more serious mental health challenges than I do. Gratitude for their friendship and ongoing concern for their well being. One of these friendships inspired the creative side of me to write a song titled "Everybody's Different," which has been developed into a play.

From my often very active creative side, many songs have been composed that relate to the topic of mental well-being. These are performed openly from time to time for various audiences.

There is even a version of "Everybody's Different" that has been performed for children, addressing the idea that everyone gets sad and what to do about it.

When the song was first introduced at a Waterford Hospital event, several professionals and parents around the room screwed up their faces as if to say, "What is Terry Rielly doing? He's going to talk to our small children about depression?"

I pride myself on being able to relate real life issues in a way that even young children can relate to. "Have you ever been sad?" I asked. We all get sad!

Confession time: I HATE taking meds! This attitude may never change, but finally I've accepted that they do make me a more pleasant person to be around and a happier "Teddy Bear Man."

One of the two medications I take regularly now was prescribed after I was tested and diagnosed with having ADD. So what came first? Did ADD complicate my life and lead to . . . or . . . whatever. Life happens!

That diagnosis is a story in itself and revealed to me at least one of the flaws in our health care system. But perhaps that is a story for another time. I have trouble focusing on more than one thing at a time and I don't want to lose my train of thought here with you about the . . . oh yeah! The depression thing.

Malcolm, my psychologist, has helped me at different times with my depression, and helped BIG TIME! Love that man.

We did have one ongoing disagreement that lasted over several sessions. He'd often ask, "So how are you doing?" and "What have you done for yourself lately?"

The problem was that when he asked about me doing something for myself, I'd talk about something done to assist someone else or some group or whatever. I really don't consider myself a goody-goody, but simply tried to convince Malcolm that one of my greatest pleasures was, and is, being helpful to others: to serve somebody in some way, be it large or small. I love to make people happy.

There's a rap song I do for family performances called "It's Cool to Care!"

Finally after one appointment, I agreed to try my best to do something before our next session that was "just for me." Something totally self-indulgent.

As chance would happen, I had to stop into the grocery store after that appointment. Seeing creamer, next to the milk, I thought, "Hey! I'm going to treat MYSELF to cream for my coffee." And did!

Somewhat proudly, I entered Malcolm's office for my next appointment. He could tell right away from the beam on my face I was pretty happy about something.

When I told him about the cream thing, he shook my hand and congratulated me. "How's it feel?" he asked, sharing in my good news.

"It was great!" I replied. "I really did enjoy it."

His expression then got serious. "Wait a minute. What do you mean 'was' and 'did'? Aren't you still buying it?"

My facial expression gave him his answer and immediately he gave me a "thumbs down" on doing something "just for me!"

Oops! He's glad to know that subsequently I've gone back to regular use of creamer — 10%; 18% when the expiry date is later than that on the 10%. Freshness is important. Right?

I do have a GREAT life, but accept that without the help of people such as doctors, supportive friends, and a loving wife, I might have continued down that long dark tunnel. And it might have got much darker. For far too many, life continues to get darker. Society has a long way to come before it knows how to help shine some light for those afraid to admit they are not well, and that it's not physical. It's mental, and there is no shame to say or even cry out, "Help me!" A recent song composed is titled, "I Am Not Well."

As much as I hate to admit, medications have become part of my everyday life. I also willingly make appointments with Malcolm as the need arises. I'm grateful that a mix of solutions was found to allow me to get on with daily life and with the joy it ought to have. Admittedly I am slow to get into a program of other alternatives. Did I say that focus is often a weak point?

Recently I'm glad to report that the recent WRAP (Wellness

Recovery Action Plan) workshop was added to my resources. It was a good one! Sort of like putting a little cream in my coffee. It's also a delight to become a CHANNAL member. What a great group of people!

I'm a much happier Teddy Bear Man most days, and much more at peace with myself. At sixty, perhaps it's time to start working on being a "wise old man."

"Everybody's Different" (6'00) 'C'

Chorus: Everybody's different, so different I'll be too,
Hope that doesn't scare you. Sorry, if I do!
I think you're very, very nice. You might be smarter too!
Some of us like to sing. What do you like to do?
Everybody's different. I think that's really GREAT!
The world would be so boring, if we were all the same.

Found out I have depression. That means that I get sad.
I couldn't understand it, 'cos I'm a very lucky man!
I get to play with children. Hang out with teddy bears!
I sing important songs, like "It's Cool To Care!"
But I do have my bad days, like most people do!
We need to have our good friends. I'm glad that I have you!

(Ch)

If we all dressed the same — wore ponytails in our hair.
If we were all Terry Riellys, it'd be more than I could bear!
Sometimes we meet somebody, who seems really different,
Little might we think, they could become our friend,
With openness to differences, you know, you just might find
A friendship you can cherish, just 'cos you took the time.

(Ch)

DEATH AND I . . . A LOVE STORY

Frances McNiven, St. John's, NL

My biggest problem is death or rather my obsession with death. Death has been a constant companion of mine for as long as I can remember. As a child of nine or ten, I remember thinking that I would die young because I could see no future for myself. As I grew older, the thought of dying young became a wish to die young. The only future I saw for myself was one of failure and disappointment. But still it was only a wish of a sad and frightened child.

I was hopeless and helpless. I had no idea how to deal with the real world, no idea how to take care of myself. But then I met my husband; he would take care of me. I was still hopeless and helpless but I was harmless. That changed when I got sick.

My mom had always said I "go from one extreme to another." Well, I guess over thirty suicide attempts could be considered extreme. People are always asking me why I was so determined to hurt myself. I have always hated myself, always wanted to hurt myself. I saw myself as weak and simple-minded, fat and useless, unworthy of life. But the fear of the pain was holding me back. Then I discovered overdoses: a way I could hurt myself, kill myself, without pain. A new obsession took hold of my mind. It chanted to me day and night. I could get no peace. I could get no respect. I was consumed with one thought and one thought only: "Destroy yourself."

Then there was the anger. A white, hot rage that would wash

over me, blinding me, making me want to rip the world apart with my bare hands. Normally a quiet and peaceful person, I was taught at an early age that anger was not "proper." I tried to contain the rage but it would build and build until I thought I would explode. Then I would take all this rage out on the only person I felt I could — myself. And my mind would scream, "You have to do something, you have to do something RIGHT now. Destroy yourself." And before I knew it, another overdose, and another stay in the hospital.

I always felt better after an overdose, happy, cheerful even. No one knew why but I think that it has something to do with lashing out. The release of some of the anger. It felt like Relief. It felt like a solution. If I could only get it "right." I would have to try again. I felt it was an endless cycle doomed to repeat itself over and over.

I had one bright, shining light on my side — my husband. My saviour, my knight in shining armour. He stood by me through the madness when I screamed that I hated him and desperately tried to push him away. He stood strong. He hid my pills over and over again, praying that this time I would not find them. This time I would not overdose. Afraid to leave me by myself for too long, determined to save me from myself, convinced that I deserved life, convinced I deserved love.

He was there at every hospital stay, visiting twice a day, every day. He was there at every doctor's appointment, asking questions, trying to understand what was wrong and how he could help me. And most importantly he was there every day and every night, my pills in his hand, just standing there until I would agree to take them. Sometimes I thought that he would stand there forever, not giving up, not backing down, determined to give me the pills that would, in his mind, save me.

Human beings are great adapters. That is what my husband did, he adapted. He got good at hiding pills, so no more overdoses! He made sure my prescriptions were filled, my pills taken every day on time, doctors' appointments kept. And not only kept but he was there making sure that I was honest with the doctor. No more hiding from my feelings. No more pretending that I was "fine."

I think my husband's only goal in life became keeping me safe, and it began to work. Bit by bit I began to understand. I had always felt that there was something wrong with me, that I was flawed somehow. That I was "bad" and "undisciplined." Slowly I began to accept that it was not "my fault" that I had an illness called bipolar disorder. It was a bit harder for me to understand because I wasn't just manic or just depressed. I was having what was called "mixed states." I was both manic — having lots of energy, not sleeping much and racing thoughts — and depressed — feeling helpless . . . hopeless . . . angry — at the same time, or as I call it, "the worst of both worlds."

Someone once said that knowledge is power. That is true. As I slowly began to understand what was wrong with me I started to get better very slowly. It took me nine hard years to get me where I am. Nine years of confusion, anger and tears. But today I am okay. It's been a year since my last overdose and for the first time in my life, I want to live. My life is not perfect. I still don't like myself very much. But there is a hope for tomorrow and that is something I am glad to give.

LONGING TO REGAIN HER LIFE

Sandra Loveless, Dartmouth, NS

For eighteen years now mental illness has been a constant factor in our family's life.

I don't remember a specific day, but over a period of time it gradually consumed my mother's life.

Diagnosed with depression and anxiety, the outgoing, lovely woman I remembered as a child slowly lost part of herself.

During the first few years we prayed and hoped that some medication would return some quality of life to her. After a while, we unwillingly realized that nothing appeared to work. Mom would go to bed for several days, feeling helpless and alone. She would cry and get upset with herself; it's the frustration of a woman who longs to regain her life.

That sense of helplessness was not restricted to Mom but was shared by the entire family. I spent many days researching mental illness and emailing health care professionals in hope that I could find a solution. Some days, it feels like we have turned a corner only to be bitterly disappointed after a few days. If we feel this way, I cannot imagine how she feels.

The effects of mental illness have a ripple effect through the entire family. Everyone seems to experience different feelings at different times. One day, someone feels angry at the disease while someone else feels dumb. As a family, we try to do our best to acknowledge her feelings and be a support system for her. Whether it be listening or trying to offer some kind of encouragement, everyone tries to do a part.

My attempts to explain how this feels to others are difficult. Some people have knowledge on the issue and are not afraid to listen and offer views; for others, they are not sure what to say or how to react, which deters me sometimes from saying anything at all to people.

Mom always tells us depression has become the reason to excuse everything in her life. If, for instance, she has a physical problem, it is not taken seriously, because if the doctor sees depression on her chart, everything she feels is attributed to that. And the physical symptoms are not acknowledged. Unfortunately, we will never know if this is a fact. This year she was diagnosed with cancer. Now things are different and suddenly depression seems to have taken a secondary role, which is not to say that it does not factor into the illness.

When we first found out about the cancer, there was concern that she might succumb to her depression by staying in bed. We feared that she would dismiss the cancer by blaming the depression for anything she felt. However, she is putting up a good fight.

Perhaps I am to blame for that fear; maybe I have not really paid attention to her symptoms and other ailments myself and blamed depression for it all. If that is the case, I am truly sorry.

Sometimes in life, you unintentionally do things that you regret later. I can say that I truly acknowledged the mental illness and attended therapy sessions with her and tried to be a great support.

The entire family loves Mom, and having depression has not changed that. It is a terrible disease and it feels like you have lost the patient at times. When she withdrew from us the pain was very difficult. I am extremely close to her and call my parents every day for a chat. The days when I couldn't talk to her were difficult.

I pray every day for a cure for mental illness. I hear stories of those who have done well on some new medication and live normal lives and I envy them. I have always wanted my mom to have her life back and for me to get my mom back.

Just like cancer, mental illness is unique to each person and not everyone responds to treatment the same or wins the battle. I just hope that one day Mom can win hers.

I JUST WANTED TO BE HEALTHY

Heather Cluney, Grand Falls-Windsor, NL

I just wanted to be healthy. That's how it all started.

I was a good student who volunteered in the community and in the church. I had a wonderful family life and great friends. I figured my life was pretty close to perfect. But then I became a teenager, and I entered a stage in life that is often accompanied by self-esteem issues and uncertainty. It was then that I realized I wanted a little something more — I wanted to be physically perfect, too. I wanted it all.

I was never overweight. As a teenager, I was probably just about right according to medical and health standards. So when my family noticed that I began to cut back on certain things like potato chips and hamburgers, they were curious about my actions. I simply explained, "I'm just trying to be healthy by watching what I eat." This answer satisfied them. After all, I had not lost any weight at this point, and I really was just "watching what I ate." This new diet made me feel great and in control of my eating and my life, so I happily kept up the routine.

Then came the elimination of certain foods from my diet. I no longer ate butter, french fries, or even the occasional chocolate bar or dessert. Not eating fatty foods for about a month allowed me to shed a few pounds. Although I did not need to lose weight, I was secretly happy about my new body. These feelings only encouraged me to eliminate more foods from my diet and continue down a destructive path. I knew I had the self-control to eat even fewer calories — and I was already eating less than my body needed. I quickly became obsessed with calorie-counting. In a journal, I recorded every single morsel of food I consumed so that I could easily keep track of my eating.

I became intent on losing even more weight, so I began to exercise vigorously every day. Nearly every day I woke up at 5:00 a.m. so that I would have time to run on the treadmill and do aerobics before school. One particular day, I even stayed home from school, pretending to be sick so that I could exercise. As soon as my mom left for work, I hopped on the treadmill, eager to burn away the few calories I had eaten for breakfast.

My extremely low food intake, combined with my rigid exercise schedule, was causing my body to gradually shut down. I stopped having my periods, I was constantly cold, and I often found it extremely difficult to get to sleep at night. I even brought a small cushion to school with me so that I could sit at my desk comfortably: it hurt to sit down because of my low weight.

My mental health was rapidly deteriorating. Depression sunk in. My thoughts became distorted. No matter how little I ate, it was always too much. No matter how much I exercised, I kept pushing myself to do more. It didn't matter how skinny I was — I was never thin enough. I often told myself, "I just want to lose five more pounds. Then I'll be happy. Then I can stop dieting." But when I reached that goal, I set another. I was never satisfied.

I recall a few times scolding myself when I ate more than 400 calories in a day. I punished myself by restricting my food intake even more the next day or running for an extra fifteen minutes on the treadmill.

I was often irritable and had frequent arguments with family members. Many times, I became upset with my parents if they purchased the wrong item at the grocery store: regular jam instead of ultra low-calorie jam or buttered popcorn instead of plain popcorn.

I recall feeling frustrated one day because my mom had brought home chewing gum that had two more calories per stick than the brand I always bought.

People around me watched as my physical and mental health took a steep decline. Some friends wondered, "Why don't you just eat something?" as if the solution were only simple. It was a far more complex problem than they understood. I recall other friends and family members trying to help me. They told me that I didn't look well and that perhaps I was taking this "healthy eating thing" a little too far. But I was not ready for help, so I became defensive when anyone suggested I see a doctor.

I would soon realize the seriousness of my condition. I remember clearly the moment I saw myself for what I had become. I had just received my school picture that had been taken a few months earlier. I was shocked by the photo. I looked severely ill, just as my family and friends had said. I'm not sure if I attributed my poor appearance to my low body weight just then. I just knew I did not look right.

The next time my mother pleaded with me to see a doctor, I reluctantly agreed. This began the healing process.

My family doctor referred me to a psychiatrist and a dietician, who played integral roles in my recovery. My psychiatrist told me that getting better would not be easy, because I suffered from a mental illness that was manifested physically. I would first need to deal with the negative thoughts, and then work on gaining weight. He helped me to untangle my distorted thoughts and change my self-image. It was a slow and painful process, mainly because of my unwillingness to change my ways. I liked being in control of my eating and in control of my life. It took me some time to realize that I really wasn't in control at all — the disease controlled me. Through counselling and with prescribed medications, I eventually rid myself of the depression that plagued my mind throughout the illness. Meanwhile, my dietician taught me the principles of *true* healthy eating and helped me to slowly increase my food intake, so that I gained some much-needed weight.

Recovery had its ups and downs. I cried when I reached 100 pounds on the scale. I felt ugly and fat. With the help of my family, friends, and medical team, I pressed on. Fortunately, recovery also delivered some benefits. I realized this fact the day I allowed myself to eat peanut butter again. Oh, how I had missed it!

I now consider myself to be fully recovered. Both my mind and body feel healthier than ever before! I have long since achieved my ideal weight. More importantly, I have learned how to value myself and I now know that self-worth is not based on body size. My personal experience with this disease has led me to pursue a career in clinical nutrition. Perhaps someday I will help someone who is struggling with disordered eating and disordered thinking to realize their own self-worth through recovery.

PRISONER IN MY OWN MIND

Cathy Melee, St. John's, NL

My counsellor today helps me with my inner child. She does that, I've learned, because of what happened to me when I was very young. My story starts with my mom. I was ten years old when she got sick. She has bipolar disorder. She has been in and out of hospital several times a year for seventeen years now. She still suffers. She had several shock treatments and has lost a lot of memories.

I used to hate it when the phone would ring early in the morning, or when she'd come home from seeing the psychiatrist. Most times she'd have to go pack her bag and leave again. It was very hard on me being the only girl in the house and having her gone. She has missed everything from birthdays to even graduation. The hardest things for me were having to say goodnight to my mom on the phone many, many times, not having her there to tuck me in at times, and when we would go visit her she wouldn't know or remember things.

I started to have anxiety at a very young age. School brought on a lot of anxiety for me too. I found it very difficult. As the grades went on my anxiety got worse. I was always, and still am, very hard and negative towards myself.

With my mom being ill and gone a lot, I tried to cope on my own. Bottling things up became my game. I just got used to keeping feelings and things inside. Then at the age of eighteen I kind of cracked.

I managed, with support, to complete high school, and I went to the College of the North Atlantic. That made things that I had bottled up come out, and drove my anxiety through the roof. The doctor suggested I leave school before I made myself really sick.

After leaving school I joined a program that was offered at the Buckmaster's Circle Community Centre. It was called Linkages. With this program I was placed to work at a daycare for nine months. When that was finished I was laid off and went on unemployment. I had a lot of time to think and my mind went into overdrive. I was crying all the time, always down and very moody. I had no idea what was going on with me so I got into drugs to self-medicate. Drugs were the quick and easy way to deal with my pain. I went from weed to pills. My parents were fed up with my moods, with me always crying, and with not knowing what was really going on with me. They took me to the doctor and that's when I was diagnosed with depression and anxiety. So I was put on medication. Also at that time neither my parents nor doctor knew I was on drugs. I couldn't tell them at this time, I was too scared. This lasted for about five months. I was 150 pounds at 5'11" and I dropped to 118 pounds. I went back to my family doctor and told her what I was doing. She then suggested that I go to the Recovery Centre. I automatically told her no and walked home. Halfway home I called my mom to pick me up and take me there. I knew I had hurt my parents by doing this, but they knew I was going to do the right thing and get help. I stayed there for seven days, got clean and went home.

Shortly after I had finished rehab I was still feeling down and really not myself. I attempted to take my life twice with my mom's pills. My mom, both times, had to bring me to hospital. I was referred to the START Clinic. That, however, did not work out for me. I didn't make any improvement.

I then got referred to see Christine Riggs. Ten minutes into our first therapy session I knew things were going to work out and that I had found the right person to help me. Being referred there to see

Christine is one of the best things that has ever happened to me. Who knows where I would be right now? At this time I was depressed and I needed someone to talk to and to give me help and guidance with my depression, anxiety and my home life. By far, words can't explain the help I got from Christine.

But then I started work again and it started to interfere with my appointments with Christine. I couldn't afford to miss work, so I had to stop my therapy sessions. At that point I thought I was doing great and I couldn't have felt better about myself. Boy was I wrong! If I had my time back I would have picked my health over my job. I guess we all learn from our mistakes.

After about six months of being back to work and away from therapy I started to hang around with a new group of friends and eventually we all got into drugs. I had relapsed, and bad this time. I was doing cocaine pretty much every day for a whole year. I had never stolen anything in my life until this; I started taking money from my parents and always lying. I'd become someone I didn't even recognize. I was disappointed in myself.

I woke up one day and started reading over the things that I had from the Recovery Centre. I was sick of what I was doing so I gave up the drugs again and stopped hanging around with the crowd I was with. I tried to continue on despite the pain of my mom being ill, my constant feelings of failure, my illness, and my past decisions. Three weeks after being clean again, I got pregnant. I was in a bad situation, but despite that, my parents supported me and stuck by my side. I was going to raise the baby on my own with my parents pushing me and encouraging me every minute.

Things felt great but really I just pushed everything aside again, and hid them in the back of my mind and heart. Being pregnant was like a little distraction. At three and a half months I had a miscarriage; I was devastated. I fell apart and all of the previous issues I had before, that I thought I had buried, came back to haunt me. I got really depressed and my anxiety went through the roof again. I wouldn't go anywhere and my parents even had to tell me to get a shower. I was a mess. I had become a prisoner in my own mind.

Then I returned to my family doctor for a check-up and she decided she was going to phone Christine to see if she could take me back on as a client. She also got me to see a psychiatrist who diagnosed me with major depressive disorder and co-morbid generalized anxiety disorder. So then I started therapy again.

I still see Christine; I see her once a week. I've been seeing her for a long time and she has helped, and helps me, deal with so much. I am learning ways of coping with my mom, my miscarriage, my illness, my home life and my inner child. This little girl has been hurting for a long time. Christine also works with me on my self-confidence, self-esteem, and encourages me to do what she knows I can. Sometimes, if I am going through a difficult period, she is there to encourage me to just keep pushing forward.

I had told Christine that I would never go back to school ever, but she helped me get into the Waterford Bridge Road Centre of the College of the North Atlantic. Now I have more supporters. My teachers, Donna, John, Jeff, Dave and Wendy, work with me very closely at school. They have encouraged me to go further into post-secondary to do welding. I have refreshed my high school math and English, and have completed several post-secondary English courses. Currently I am doing other post-secondary courses in math and customer services. This is part of the bridging program to Prince Philip Drive where I will go in September to do welding. I will have all the related academic courses completed upon my arrival, so I will not have the anxiety of a full course load, and can concentrate on the practical part of the course.

I am now working with an amazing group of different health care workers. On my team I have my therapist, family doctor, psychiatrist, teachers, and parents. Because we all work together all my needs are being met. Communication with team members has resulted in a new diagnosis. It has been determined that I have bipolar spectrum disorder, and soon I will be starting new medication. I'm in a much better place now then ever before. I still have a long road ahead of me, but with all my supporters and my new belief in myself I'm headed down the right path.

THE MENTAL HEALTH OF A TOXIC WORKPLACE

Anonymous

The Toxic Workplace. My toxic workplace is not a workplace that is toxic because of chemicals, hazardous materials, and processes carried out at the work site, but rather is a workplace that has become toxic due to human interactions at the site. The ingredients for our toxic workplace include micromanagement, ineffective supervision, complacency, no defined purpose, a stagnant work force and little room for advancement. The effects of this toxic combination are employee disengagement, high sick leave usage, conflict between employees, increased customer service complaints, the existence of cliques, low morale and poor mental health of many, if not all, employees at the site.

It has been a number of years now since I moved to a workplace that I would come to describe as toxic. It didn't take long at the new site to conclude that something was wrong, terribly wrong. Sick leave usage was rampant, most people who came to work did so for a cheque rather than for an organizational purpose. At one point about 20% of the workforce was on long-term sick leave. There were frequent confrontations between employees. Some conflicts between employees had raged for years, cliques existed, social events were nonexistent, teamwork was absent, complaints by customers were frequent and morale was in the toilet. Emotion was often released through tears, words and actions. There was little ownership evident, work stations were a mess and the lunchroom and offices were always in need of attention.

A number of employees recognized the severity of the problem and individually, worked hard towards improvement. Despite valiant efforts, improvement did not emerge. As I came to be known at the new site as a dedicated, hard-working person who cared about people, some people started to open up to me. The stories they told confirmed that we worked at a toxic workplace and our "boss" was a micromanager.

Stress and stress-related illness were all around. The employee assistance program (EAP) was accessed by many employees. But why, I often wondered, didn't the employer deal with the situation? Apparently the employer was well aware of the situation; reports had been written and consultants had been consulted with. The union had been involved and complaints had been filed. Could it be that they didn't care? I don't think so. As I pondered this issue the only conclusion that made sense to me was that they did not understand the gravity of the situation. They did not understand the adverse health (mental) effects of the situation. They were ill prepared to deal with the situation. Does that let an employer, particularly an employer who operates on tax dollars, off the hook? Absolutely not!

It is the responsibility of all employers to learn about stress in the workplace and its health effects. Early intervention, accommodation, support and understanding are what's needed. They practice these things now for physical health. Think of the employee who breaks a leg playing hockey. The employer is very understanding, the employer will encourage an early return to work, perhaps the employer will modify the work station or work schedule. All this without hesitation. Why is the employer's approach to mental health different?

The Mental Health Damage. The mental health damage resulting from this situation is far reaching. Many employees required care from their family doctor and other health care professionals such as counsellors, psychologists and psychiatrists. The negative mental health effects upon the employees spilled over to their families and friends. It affected work, productivity and customer service.

On a personal note, I did not escape the damage. On a particular day during a confrontation with my micromanager boss, I felt my stress level escalate to the point where I experienced significant pain and discomfort in my chest. I immediately reported off sick and made arrangements to see my family doctor. Blood tests and diagnostics were used in rapid fashion. Diagnosis: significantly high and chronic stress causing health problems. I accessed a counsellor through EAP and we worked through a plan for me to stay in that toxic workplace, but only until I was eligible for early retirement.

All employees survived this toxic workplace exposure but some will be affected forever. Five employees took early retirement, very early retirement. A number of others moved from the area or transferred to other departments. Most were good employees. They were very good workers but they didn't work as well with a mental health injury! The total damage caused by the situation was huge. The sad thing is that most of the damage was preventable.

Talk is not sufficient. Most public employers communicate a respectful workplace policy, but words alone are insufficient. Words are cheap. Action and change are required. Action is not cheap and change is always a challenge. Both require strong leadership and a significant investment of money and people. Regardless of the cost for action and change, does it not outweigh the cost of the damage to the employees and their families?

Stress-related illness in the workplace is real, Its effects can be severe. Denial is no longer an accepted response. Action is required.

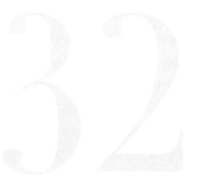

MY LIFE

Anonymous

I was born the son of Mike, the kind of kid everyone seemed to like. It just seemed my life just felt like a dream. What ever happened? I did not care. Everything seemed so unfair. I was quite a shy boy without much to say but it didn't matter anyway. In my teens I went through school always acting like a fool.

One thing, it did not matter: a speeding car with no brake pedal. The one day as I laughed, my body just ran out of gas. I went to see a doctor to see what was wrong. "You're a sick young man." I did not belong.

I was an outpatient for many years and my eyes could not hold back the tears. Life went by in a state of fear. I hid my illness from everyone: my brother, my sister, everyone. The first year diagnosed was the roughest and I was determined to be the toughest. All through the night I would be praying to God to let me live.

The first three and a half years were the roughest and I was determined to become the toughest. I drank, partied and yelled. I could not break Satan's spell. I prayed and prayed my heart out: "Please help me, leave me." In May 1985, after having depression from the age of twelve, God rescued me from my personal hell. I have basically been pretty well rescued from my hell. Each day was hard, never easy. Most of my life has been pretty creepy. Today I am feeling pretty well. I married, built a house, and we live by ourselves with two cats. My advice is never quit; get referred for help. Then take this disease, take a sledgehammer and break its two knees.

THE HIDDEN CHAPTER

Suzanne Emberley Peddle, St. John's, NL

Everyone has stories they carry throughout their lives. What we do with these stories is our choice. One can tell them or can hide them — but they cannot be changed. For a long time I did not share a chapter of my story because it did not fit into the image I wanted to portray to the world. I thought others might define me by this one aspect of my life, as if all other positive attributes would be cancelled out.

I am a twenty-eight-year-old woman. I have a successful occupation, a husband, a house, and a dog. I am a contributing member of society: I am also someone with a mental illness. My struggle with anxiety and depression began when I was about fifteen years old. At the age when most teenagers are impulsive and rebellious, I was all those things in addition to being depressed and anxious. For a long time my behaviour was chalked up to teenage rebellion, until it became apparent there was something else going on. I was more than sad; I was crying most days, couldn't sleep, and was constantly nervous. The things that had always brought joy to my life no longer did.

I reluctantly began seeing a psychiatrist and a psychologist, as well as starting to take antidepressants. I was having severe panic attacks and debilitating depression. My psychiatrist tried me on several medications, none of which proved to be effective. This went on for over a year, at which point my behaviour continued to spiral downward.

I was distraught, so sad that I could feel it physically, like something was breaking inside me. I became suicidal; I didn't want to die but life had become unbearable. At seventeen, I could no longer function and had to be hospitalized. I remember feeling relieved at first and feeling that, at the very least, things would change. People now clearly saw how I was feeling and there was no hiding it any longer, but any relief I felt quickly turned to shame. I think everything about me — my age, my personality, and my life experiences up until that point — cultivated the perfect environment for shame to flourish and grow.

I had never known anyone who talked openly about having a mental illness. There was never a point at which I felt it was "okay" to be mentally ill; therefore, it came naturally for me to hide it and try to conceal it. Only a few family members and friends were made aware of my situation. I led everyone else to believe physical ailments were responsible for my sudden drop off the face of the earth.

During my hospitalization I was given new medications which resulted in a rapid weight gain: an unpleasant side effect which didn't do much for my plummeting self-esteem. I felt numb, as if I was merely existing. I was released from the hospital but was unable to cope. Admitted and released, admitted and released: so began the revolving door. At this point my psychiatrist told me she could see my life going one of two ways: my life could become an endless series of admissions to the hospital or I could try to take positive steps and see where that led me. At the time, it almost seemed like a dare or a challenge. I guess she struck a chord in me; I chose the latter. I agreed to go to the outpatient day program at the Health Sciences Centre. I started to make better choices and learned healthier coping skills.

After I completed the program I continued to struggle but things began to look up. I managed to get my high school diploma, got a job, and started going out again. This meant one thing in my mind: I was cured! I thought that maybe there had been nothing wrong with me in the first place and I had been done a great injustice by being placed in the psychiatric ward. If there was a "do it yourself" cure for depression, I was going to find it. I didn't want to have a mental illness; I just couldn't accept it. So I embarked on the ultimate quest to cure myself: I stopped taking my medications, thought positively, and read self-help books. I heard exercise could cure depression, so I walked from one end of St. John's to the other. Nothing helped; I still had that feeling of dread — a dark cloud following me everywhere I went. Needless to say, things didn't go exactly how I planned, and before long I was once again in the midst of a major depression. It finally began to register with me that I had an illness, and like any illness it could not be willed away: it had to be treated.

Feeling defeated, I agreed to try yet another new antidepressant, and for the first time something actually worked for me. The medication didn't drastically change how I was feeling but it lessened the severity of my symptoms, which made life liveable again. Since then, I've lived a good life. Every now and then I will have a bad day, even a bad week, but I wait — and it passes. I feel I am not so different from anyone else dealing with everyday life in that regard.

Despite the mental health issues I struggle with, even in the darkest moments of my life, I always had a glimmer of hope. Hope that I could have something more and that I was bigger than the things that were happening to me: it just took a long time for me to believe this.

So here I am years later and I'm finally ready to be open and honest about this chapter in my story. I used to think that being able to walk down the street without everyone knowing your life and your story was freedom — except I never felt free. I always felt that I was disregarding parts of my life and tearing out pages of my story. I was trying to rewrite my life and make it into something else. Something I could accept and that would be more readily accepted by society.

It took me a long time, but I am finally beginning to feel free from the shame I associated with having a mental illness. I still have fear that my life could go on that downward slope and I could end up back where I was years ago. However, fear I can live with: shame I cannot.

So, the secret is out: I have a mental illness. It's the part of my life that has caused me incredible grief, agony, denial, and shame. It is the story I could never tell. But just as you cannot live your life giving half of who you are or being half yourself — you can't tell half of your story. Hopefully someone else struggling with a mental illness can relate to my story; it could even help them in some way. Maybe they won't waste as much time as I have fighting to accept it and feeling ashamed of it. I know by writing that part of my story I have helped at least one person: myself.

FROM DEATH TO LIFE

Anonymous

I was dead.

I couldn't be dead though. I was breathing, walking, talking. But I felt dead. Just to be sure, I ran the blade across my skin to see if I would bleed. After all, dead people don't bleed. Blood. Bright red and gushing. Sure enough, I was alive. But if I was alive, why did I feel so dead?

Life was going pretty well — at least on paper it was. I had two undergraduate degrees, a promising career, a loving family, and great friends. On paper, I had it all. Inside, I had nothing. I guess I always knew that something wasn't right, but it wasn't until 2004 at the age of twenty-three that someone else noticed. I was sitting in my apartment with a variety of pills lined up on the coffee table. I wasn't afraid to die. I was already dead. I started taking them one by one, washing them down with mouthfuls of beer, when a friend walked in. She had suspected that something was wrong and her gut instinct proved to be right. She sat with me through the night and then insisted I go see my family doctor the next day.

Bipolar disorder. That was the diagnosis made by my family doctor which was later confirmed by a psychiatrist. I was placed on a combination of medications to help me cope.

I'm an educated person and now that I had the diagnosis, I learned what I could about the disorder. The more I read, the more

I kept thinking to myself, "I don't have bipolar disorder." But what did I know? I wasn't a doctor. Months went by and the medication didn't seem to help. I finally had had enough of pumping my body full of medication without any improvement. I went to another doctor and requested to be taken off all medication. He listened to me and wondered if I was suffering from depression. He referred me to a different psychiatrist and recommended a psychologist and I went to see her with very few expectations and a bit of an attitude.

I guess I can't really blame the doctors. They didn't have all the information.

Much to my surprise, I developed an excellent counselling relationship with my psychologist, and within a couple of months I felt comfortable enough to share what I had held inside for so long.

I was raped. I was fifteen at the time and under the influence of large amounts of alcohol. I guess I always blamed myself, but she got me to see the situation for what it really was. I also disclosed that I had been sexually abused when I was eight years old. For so long I thought there was something wrong with me. Why else would it happen twice to the same person? The only common denominator was me.

I was given a new diagnosis: post-traumatic stress disorder. When I started researching this diagnosis, I got scared. It was as if the signs and symptoms of this disorder were written based on me: exposure to traumatic event — check; persistent re-experience — check; persistent avoidance of stimuli associated with the trauma — check; persistent symptoms of increased arousal — check; duration of symptoms more than one month — check; significant impairment in social, occupational, or other important areas of functioning — check. I knew that this time they were right. I grieved this diagnosis. I didn't want to fit a label, but at the same time I was relieved to finally have something that could explain how I had felt all these years.

I've come a long way since that night in 2004. I have gone on to finish a graduate degree in counselling psychology and now work within the education system. I have gotten married and hope to start a family soon. I have also come a long way in terms of coping strategies and no longer abuse alcohol or drugs, and cutting is no longer a part of my regular routine. The physical scars are still there, but I consider them daily reminders of how far I have come.

The emotional scars are still there too. I still struggle. I am constantly battling depression and anxiety, and was on medication for a while to help with that. I have been off medication for over a year now, but still find that every day is a struggle. I have nightmares, I'm constantly on guard, and I can sometimes be withdrawn, but I'm getting there. I still see my psychologist on a regular basis and she helps me tremendously. Above all else, I feel as if I'm moving forward and that is what matters most to me.

My story doesn't end here. My story has many more chapters to go and I look forward to every one of them because each new chapter means I'm alive.

I'm alive.

HOPE THROUGH THE DARKNESS

Shirley Gosse, St. John's, NL

I was a young child in grade school when the teacher strapped me until my hands bled. I remember the teacher got me to read in front of the class so that the students would make fun of me. I had a speech problem and I think that was the reason he was picking on me. When I got 80% or 90% in a test, for example geography or language, he used to take me up by the ears and say, "Shirley, you're stupid." I would go back to my desk and cry; what could I say back to a teacher? After I heard the word "stupid" for a year, I started to believe that I was stupid. I used to stay in my room as a child, crying myself to sleep each night and saying to myself, "Oh God, why am I so stupid?" When I was eleven years old, I got hold of my grandmother's pills and took them, but it did no harm because they weren't strong enough. I remember Mom looked everywhere for Grandmother's pills but could not find them. Mom never did know that I took them.

As a teenager I spent most of my time crying and wondering why I was so different from everyone else. At the age of sixteen I quit school and went to work in a fish plant. Things got worse because I let myself be abused physically and sexually, and I thought I deserved it. At the age of nineteen I became pregnant. My son was born in 1974. That was the best thing that happened to me; it gave me a reason to go on living. After I had my son I went to live with my parents in a small community in Bay d'Espoir. At that time society was not open-minded, and unwed mothers were frowned upon. This was very hurtful.

For the first two years I built my life around my son. And my friend Della encouraged me to return to school and I received my grade eleven diploma. Everything was going well for me until my son's father came back into my life. I'm not going to go into any details about what happened, but negative things entered my life again.

I was twenty-two when I suffered a severe depression and ended up in hospital. I remember the doctor put me on lots of drugs; I felt high and I was enjoying the feeling. After I was discharged and left the "safety" of the hospital there were lots of times I pretended that I was sick so that I would have to go back to the hospital. I was really good at making the doctors believe that I was sick. I was diagnosed with many different kinds of mental illness at the time such as manic depressive, with a bipolar disorder. After seven years of going back and forth to hospital, the doctor realized what I was doing and he told me it wasn't possible for me to be admitted to hospital whenever I was unable to face the negative atmosphere within the community.

It was New Year's Eve and another year was about to begin. There was no change so I tried to overdose on pills. The sad thing was that my son watched me and he started to cry. He was ten years old at the time. My mom phoned the ambulance and got me to the hospital. That was where I met Doctor Nurse, who became a very positive influence in my life. He was a very caring man and took the time to listen to what I had to say. He took me off most of the medications and told me I didn't need them. He told me I needed to get away from the community I was living in. He sent me to St. John's to a place called Emmanuel House, a "safe house" for people with difficulties in their lives who needed a place to stay for the short-term. I didn't have a clue at the time what kind of place it was. But I knew I had to get away, because if I didn't, I would mess up my son's life. I remember I wanted to protect my son no matter what kind of place it was. I don't remember how I got to Emmanuel House in the state of mind I was in. I remember when I arrived at Emmanuel House I looked at the taxi driver and said that I was scared and he went in with me. I will always remember how kind the taxi driver was, how he comforted me when he knew that I was scared. I will never forget his kind face.

At first when I went to Emmanuel House, the only thing I wanted to do was to commit suicide. I spent a lot of time trying to figure out what time and when. After I was at Emmanuel House a while, things changed. I began to see counsellors at the Waterford Hospital. They spent lots of time with me and so did the counsellors at Emmanuel House. With so much support I realized that people did care about me and I began to have hope for the first time in my life.

I met a wonderful man, who was also at Emmanuel House for addiction issues. He fell in love with me. It took me a long time before I could trust and accept his love. I did everything to turn him against me but nothing worked; years later we got married. After we got married I went to work at Jack and Jill home care. I worked with Jack and Jill home care for three years before I got pregnant. After I got pregnant I had to stay at home because working with Jack and Jill involved lots of lifting and I was afraid of miscarriage. My first daughter was born in 1990. After that I went back to work. I only worked for a couple of weeks when I found out I was pregnant again. My first daughter was two months old; my second daughter was born in 1991. After that I stayed at home to raise my family. We found it very difficult because only my husband worked. We had to struggle to get by. We managed because we had lots of support from family and friends. It was never easy for me to be married and raise a family with my illness.

When my children got older I began to feel useless; I got sick again. For a while I thought I was going to lose everything that I worked so hard for. I knew that I put my husband and children through a lot at that time. I began to lose hope again and I just wanted to give up. Then I heard about the recycling program at Mill

Lane. I went to the program and with the support from the staff, I came a long way. Working at Mill Lane made me realize lots of things about myself. It made me realize I wasn't a bad person and I wasn't "stupid." For years I was hard on myself for being no good. Working around people with mental illness made me realize what your mind can do to you. For the first time in my life I had a chance to be happy, but my mind wouldn't let me. When I thought I was going to have a nervous breakdown, the support from the staff really helped me get through it. I realized also that I missed a lot in life because of what my mind was telling me.

Because of the support I received while working with the recycling program I now can let go of the past and get on with my life. My mind is finally relaxed. Right now I have everything you could ask for: a good husband, two wonderful daughters, and a wonderful son. Thank God, right now I can enjoy them. I still have to work hard at staying well, going for walks and other activities to keep my mind occupied, because if I don't, I will end up sick again. All the fighting I have done to make my life better is now starting to pay off. Right now I am happy to be alive.

DEALING WITH STIGMA ASSOCIATED WITH MENTAL ILLNESS

Anonymous

For the past forty-one years, I've been living with a mental illness, specifically obsessive-compulsive disorder, (generally referred to as OCD). I'm a fifty-one-year-old male resident of St. John's, born and raised in the city, who first noticed some of the symptoms of the disorder while I was an elementary school student. While some people with OCD have obsessive thoughts (such as an unnatural fear of the death of a loved one), others like myself display some type of obsessive behaviour. In my case, the unusual behaviour took the form of excessive hand-washing, as well as performing little "rituals" throughout the day. I clearly remember the morning routine I just HAD to go through each day before leaving for school. This included re-arranging the cushions on the living room sofa, straightening the ornaments on the mantle, and making sure that all the labels of food items in our pantry faced outward! I also was overly concerned about how my clothes were stored and how books were arranged on shelves and bookcases.

My parents may have liked having a kid who wasn't a slob, but this sometimes led to friction with my two younger brothers. We shared the same bedroom for several years as children, with many common areas such as the clothes closet, bookcase, and a desk to use for homework. As you can imagine, my policy of "a place for everything and everything in its place" didn't go over very well, especially within the confines of a small and sometimes cluttered room! Despite all this, I managed to do well at school, graduating from Brother Rice High in June of 1974 and entering Memorial University that fall. After losing a year because of a change in my course of study, I finished my degree program in 1979 with a Bachelor of Arts, majoring in political science.

Around this time, the symptoms of OCD stepped up dramatically, especially around the ritual behaviour I had to go through at the start of each day. In addition to the "tidy up the house" routine, I became fixated on having to complete EVERYTHING to perfection. This included such everyday tasks as washing, dressing, and especially shaving. During my worst periods, I could often spend several hours each day on these "routine" chores, a problem made even more acute in a one-bathroom house for a family of six! By 1984, I had (reluctantly) started seeing a psychiatrist who prescribed some pills to help diminish the ritual behaviour. The following year, that doctor left the province, reassigning my case to a colleague who urged me to consider hospitalization as a way to finally deal with the ever more powerful rituals, which by this time were ruling (and ruining) my life! It took another thirty months before I finally agreed to be admitted to the psychiatry unit at St. Clare's hospital, where I was a patient from July to September of 1988. Working with a team of doctors, nurses, psychologists and other professionals, I was able to finally reduce and to later largely eliminate the behaviour rituals that had been such a strong (and negative!) influence on my life for so many years!

Unfortunately for me, once I was discharged and left the controlled surroundings of the hospital ward, many of my OCD symptoms returned, although not as strong as before my admission. The medical staff, my family, and I all agreed that some form of supportive housing environment might be helpful to reinforce and maintain the progress already made, so I moved into ACCESS House in November of 1988. A few months later, I enrolled in a program designed to help mental health consumers obtain and maintain employment by developing skills necessary in the workplace. In my case punctuality was one of the most important! It felt very satisfying to leave ACCESS each morning, walk to the nearest bus stop in time to make the right connection, and show up at the workplace before the start of my shift.

After completing this program in June of 1989, I was hired three months later by the local office of the Canadian Mental Health Association under a funding arrangement with the provincial government. In those days before the Internet's popularity, most of my duties involved organizing, updating and maintaining CMHA's Resource Library of books and videotapes. The office was kept quite busy handling requests for information about a wide variety of mental health problems and conditions, often from family members who had no idea why their loved one's behaviour had so suddenly changed.

By the following summer, I was ready to move from the supportive housing environment of ACCESS to living in my own apartment; and that's when I found out first-hand just how unfair and hurtful stigma and prejudice are in our society. I had responded to a newspaper ad for a furnished basement apartment in a house off Freshwater Road in the city. The owner/landlord showed me around, and seemed quite eager for me to move in right away, even offering extra perks such as cable TV and use of a snow blower at no extra charge! I liked the place, and agreed to move in that weekend; so I paid the first month's rent plus a damage deposit. He issued a receipt, and we shook hands, with the owner promising to have the rental agreement drawn up and ready to be signed within twenty-four hours. Early the next morning, the landlord phoned the CMHA and left a message with the office manager for me to return the call. When I did, I was told that the apartment was no longer for rent since the man's daughter was returning to the province unexpectedly and would need a place to live. He made arrangements to return the money already paid, but gave no indication when the apartment might become available. His telephone manner was noticeably less friendly than the previous day, but I assumed that he was preoccupied by concern over his daughter's problems.

Although disappointed about losing out on the apartment, I attributed the situation to bad timing or hard luck, and continued the search. Three weeks later, I happened to be in the drugstore on the corner of Empire Avenue and Freshwater Road, only a short distance away from the residence that nearly had become my address! The quickest walking route back to ACCESS meant passing in front of the house, and since I was curious to see the place again, that's what I did. While fully expecting the "FOR RENT" sign to have been removed from the basement window, I was surprised to see three men sitting in lawn chairs near the entrance drinking beer! Being a friendly sort, I said hello and asked if any of the apartments were vacant. One of the guys, who looked to be no older than twenty, said that he had just recently moved into the basement unit and that his two buddies had stopped by for a visit. Since I had been told by the landlord that his daughter was supposed to be living there, I pressed my luck and asked how he had gotten that apartment, mentioning that I had been interested as well. He told me that when he initially contacted the landlord three weeks before, he was told that the apartment had just been rented to a guy — ME — who was going to move in that weekend. Two days after that, the owner phoned, explaining that the tenant who was going to move in had backed out, and offered to arrange a viewing!

Since I was the first tenant, and did no such thing, my first reaction was anger! "How could that so & so landlord change his mind so quickly?" And just as important: "WHY?" Checking with the office manager again, she recalled that when she answered the phone with the regular greeting of "Good Morning! Canadian Mental Health Association, Newfoundland Division," the landlord initially thought he had dialled a wrong number and asked that the name be repeated. Only when he was sure that I did actually work there did he realize that he had the right place! Thinking back to my first meeting with the owner, when he had asked where I worked, my reply was "the CMHA on Water Street." (I used the abbreviation instead of the full title!) Whether or not he confused the initials with those of the CMHC (Canada Mortgage and Housing Corporation) or some similar company, I'll probably never know. However I do know that he was caught in a lie, and that the lying started after he found out I was with an agency with the words "Mental Health" in its name!

One of the many disturbing things about this incident is how everyone connected with the mental health care system seems to have been smeared by the same brush — that we're all "nut cases." My prospective landlord didn't seem to make a distinction between the educational and advocacy functions carried out by the CMHA staff and the treatment of patients in a hospital setting. His actions seemed to follow along the lines that all "crazy" people stick together and that he didn't want one as his tenant! Nearly twenty-two years later, that condemnation by a man who barely knew me still hurts. It was one of the reasons why I became so involved with the mental health support group CHANNAL, which was just getting started at the time. The CMHA also invited consumers to participate in its own STOP STIGMA campaign, arranging visits to schools to educate both students and teachers. These sessions included information about the types of disorders (including OCD!), dispelling some of the myths surrounding mental illness and allowing the students to see for themselves that people living with mental health problems could actually do that — live with the problems, but still have useful and meaningful lives too!

Even though more laws are now on the books to prevent discrimination against people with disabilities, attitudes seem to change much more slowly! Progress is being made, but sometimes only at a snail's pace. Affordable housing remains a major problem for Canadians with low income, including mental health consumers. I can't help but wonder how many other landlords are still out there, as inflexible and close-minded as the one I encountered!

UP FROM ROCK BOTTOM

Sherri O'Halloran, Mount Pearl, NL

The day that I heard the words "you are depressed" changed my life forever. On the outside looking in I was the picture of perfection; on the inside I was fighting the demons that held me back from being the person that I used to be.

It should have been the happiest time of my life: I had a wonderful husband, two beautiful boys and was pregnant with our third baby boy. I woke every morning with a plan of action, to try my best to hide the pain that I was feeling. I played with our boys, cleaned our home, put meals on the table and a big fat fake smile on my face. No one had any idea as to what was really going on in my head. I would tell myself that it was "normal" to be feeling this way. I mean, after all, I was pregnant and just figured that it was the hormones making me feel horrible. I would eventually start feeling better, and I just thought that no one cared or had the time to "help" me. It wasn't until I broke down in my doctor's office that I realized that something was seriously wrong. I spent three days in the hospital to get started on medication, and to rest. I told my family that I was there for high blood pressure, and when I left with my new prescription I left even more determined to hide the truth. I couldn't imagine telling my family and friends that I had depression: that would be wrong for me to have something like that.

Two months later, I gave birth to a healthy baby boy. On cloud nine is where I would tell you that I was; in a deep dark hole that I couldn't get out of is where I really was. Even though I was taking my medication, it wasn't enough. I fell deeper as the days went by. I tried to get out to do things to make myself feel better but a simple trip to the drugstore was a scary experience that I will never forget. I remember walking around with a feeling that people were staring at me, and no matter where I went these people were following me, talking about me. But why? What was going on? I felt somehow threatened, so I ran out of there as fast as I could. I would spend nights up alone thinking that my family could do better than me, that if I just ran away they would be happier without me. I felt that I didn't deserve happiness. I completely shut the outside world out of my life. I only saw people when they would come visit me, and screened my phone calls. I would joke to my sister that I was going to get rid of our dog and even had a plan all worked out of how I was going to do it. She would tell me that it wasn't funny to speak about those things, and when she would ask what was going on, I would just shrug it off. The day that our then five-year-old son told me to stay on the couch and rest while he made lunch for himself and his brothers opened my eyes. I knew that I had to get more help. I got in touch with my family doctor and that day I ended up in the short-stay unit at the Waterford.

It was the worst three days of my life. I now call it my "blessing in disguise." Postpartum. But, I felt that I didn't belong there. As soon as people hear the word "postpartum" they assume the worst. I was automatically placed in a category with mothers who harm their children. Why were these people thinking this of me? And they were medical professionals. As I sat there crying, listening to them go on and on, a light bulb went off in my head. I was better than this disease; my children and husband deserved to have me. I deserved to have the best of me that I knew was there somewhere, lost in the sickness that tore my life apart. I then decided to take any help, any medication, they had to offer.

Two days later I walked through the doors of the Early Psychosis

Program at the Waterford. It was there that I met an amazing team that has helped make me the person that I am now. I was not judged; the team was there for me no matter what the case. I had someone that came to my home to check on me, and when I talked they listened. I felt comfort in knowing that someone was on my side with no strings attached. It was hard work; I didn't get better overnight, but as each day passed by, that fake smile was becoming real. I didn't have to put on a disguise to get me through the day. I also started telling other people about my experience with depression, and when people squirmed when I said those dreaded words "the Waterford" I let them know that it's okay. I am fine.

January 2009 marks fours years since I hit rock bottom. As I look back I wonder where the time went. Those days seem so far away as I look at my life now. I have learned that it's okay to ask for help; I need to take care of myself before I can take care of my family. I eat right, exercise daily and can sleep like a baby. I just recently lost close to one hundred pounds, and this summer I ran my first Tely 10 road race. Those are things that I do for me, and my family couldn't have been prouder. It's sad to think that there was a time when I was so ashamed to tell anyone that I was sick; I even thought that my husband would leave me. Thankfully he stood by me and has been my rock through it all. My wish is that one day people can come forward before it's too late and admit that they have a mental illness. People have to realize that just because you can't see it doesn't mean it's not there. I believe that with the right education and support from our doctors, family, friends and communities we can change the way any mental illness is perceived. We can rise above and I am living proof.

WALK THROUGH THE DARK

Anonymous

When I was a young boy, I always felt different but did not know why. When I felt depressed I would lock myself in my room and would not come out for days. I guess I had an illness then and that was my way of controlling it. I never had much of a childhood. I was picked on by my so-called friends in the neighbourhood. The only way to get them to stop beating me was to steal from my dad and pay the kids off, and in return my father would beat me for stealing his money.

My relationship with my father was a strange one: the only time I got along with my dad was when he was drinking. When he was sober he would beat me with his belt. I wore his belt for a long time after he died until one fateful night when I tried to strangle myself with the belt. After that I ended up at St. Clare's hospital for a month on the psychiatric unit.

My relationship with my mom was a good one. I do feel guilty because there were things going on in my life that my mom kept from my dad, which must have been stressful for her. My dad gave my mom a hard time, which was another reason I didn't like him. No physical abuse but a lot of mental abuse. I was failing in school and my dad didn't know anything. My mom knew but she just didn't tell my dad. Sometimes I blame myself for her getting sick and having a stroke because of all the stress she went through hiding things from my dad. I think my relationship with my mom is why I find it so much easier to confide in a woman more so than a man. I think my life would be easier if I had a woman for a psychiatrist.

Growing up, before I was diagnosed with schizophrenia, I always knew there was something wrong with me. I would sit for hours and stare openly into deep nothingness. Not thinking or looking at anything. I was always withdrawn from so-called life. I never really had friends; my imagination was my best friend growing up.

When I was younger, I had an interest in hockey and I was told by my coach that I would go far. I scored the most goals on my team but I was the worst skater, and my coach told me if I worked on my skating I could be a great hockey player. Then came marijuana, which screwed up my life and made me lose total interest in hockey. And to this day sometimes I get depressed when I'm watching a hockey game, realizing that I could be out there playing — yes, I was that good! The drugs made me more paranoid than my illness did. I found drugs were an escape from my reality and my illness. For ten years I smoked marijuana every day, and 95% of the time it would make me paranoid. If someone glanced at me a certain way I would think that person was out to get me. This person could be any age; it could even be a child.

When I was ill, sometimes I felt immortal. There were times when I would walk out in front of traffic not fearing for my life because I was on a natural high. Other times something as simple as my shoelace coming undone would send me into a depression. A band once said that "The Mind is a Terrible Thing to Taste" which rings very true for me. The only thing I find that gets me through the day is music — my Saviour. I could be feeling down and then I would hear a specific song that would bring me around. And yet there are other times when I would hear a song that reminded me of a time in my life when I was sick, and it would bring me right back to that moment when I was ill-tasting, feeling, hearing — all my senses on fire. Even though music was my saviour, it was also sometimes a demon. I would spend $30-$60 a week on cds — just to return them a few days later for less than $4 each, and that cycle would go on for years and it's only lately I am overcoming this part of my illness. I would get my fix and when the music didn't work for me anymore I would get rid of the cds, sometimes I would even throw them into a mailbox. Why? I don't know. Sometimes I think there's a mail carrier out there with a huge music collection, compliments of me.

Another aspect of my illness was taking on personalities of other people. If I read in a magazine about a certain individual who had similar characteristics, I would think I was becoming that person.

Another part of my illness is counting, which I'm doing right now as I am writing. I count in multiples of three; for example the word illness has seven letters in it; seven is not a multiple of three so therefore illness is not important. Cancer has six letters, so therefore cancer is important. People say when they talk about themselves to someone who cares they find their illness lessens, but with me when I talk to someone about my illness I find my illness worsens. That is why I keep things to myself, which in the end I know is worse than talking to someone. I have to learn to deal with my illness so I can take better control of my life.

There were times in my life when my illness didn't bring me down. I received a certificate in Sales and Marketing in the early 90s. That was a 36-week program where I went to school for 18 weeks and did job training for another 18 weeks. During my sales and marketing program, I worked at CHMR at the university. I had my own show Sunday nights from 1 a.m. to 3 a.m. I called my show *Adventures in the Tickle Trunk*. I also did classical music shows in the morning while I was there. At the time, I was also going to night school and working three nights a week at Wal-Mart. I found that keeping myself busy, I wouldn't think so much about my illness. I also went to university for a semester. I took four courses: English, arts, French, and philosophy. I ran into some personal problems so I had to leave. At the time I quit university, my philosophy teacher actually called my home looking for me, telling my mom that I was a gifted student and that I should come back. I really enjoyed philosophy. When I first started philosophy I think I was trying too hard to understand it. My professor told me to simplify it, which I did. I used to go to the professor's office between classes, drink coffee, and talk about philosophy. I sometimes found myself in the university bar doing school work. I would go there in the afternoon and the next thing I knew they were dimming the lights and getting ready for the evening parties. I was that engulfed in my school work.

I suffer from schizophrenia, a debilitating disease that makes me paranoid and delusional. They tried many drugs on me until I found Clozapine, which I call the last chance drug, and it works for me. I have been on this medication for twenty to twenty-five years and it seems to be working for me. I go to school full-time at the College of the North Atlantic (Adult Basic Education) and I'm also taking guitar lessons once a week, so life is getting better. I plan to take some kind of course at the College of the North Atlantic to better myself and get a good job. Right now I'm in a healthy relationship with someone who also suffers from schizophrenia and we are both getting through it together. So, remember, you have to walk through the dark to get to the light.

PUSHING MY WAY BACK

Paul Stride, St. John's, NL

> *God only knows, what takes a petal from the rose*
> *What makes the dark rivers overflow*
> *What makes a lifetime come and go*
>   Ron Hynes — "Godspeed"

It was a typical Friday night in September. The fall air had crossed some imaginary isthmus, pushing summer memories into the recesses of my mind. I drove aimlessly around the city, contemplating a life scarred by mental illness. Time had run ahead of my perceptions . . . I was in my early forties, broke, a failed marriage and careers, and nothing to show from years of hard work but traces of useless regret. Like so many in society, I was one illness away from disaster. And that night, my thoughts had culminated upon hearing the news that my insurer had turned down my disability application. I felt a sense of hopelessness never before experienced. That night, I wanted to take my own life. How did I get to that point?

In retrospect, I had been suffering from varying degrees of depression practically all my life. Officially, it started nearly ten years ago during a number of visits to my family doctor and psychologist. It was a busy year working for an employer who was going through a merger, and waiting for my middle management position to be terminated. As outgoing president of the local chamber of commerce, there were extra untold hours in service to the business community, and with it, extra stress. While craving an oasis at home, my marriage was falling apart at the same pace as my health.

Reluctantly, my doctor prescribed an antidepressant. Close friends, not understanding the illness, strongly suggested I not take "pills." Other acquaintances chose to break contact rather than confront what they saw as awkward. In the middle of a situation that offered no holistic approach, there was stigma to worry about. Finding a balance between privacy and honesty was difficult. My illness was not obvious like a broken bone or recovery from surgery. Many had questions about a person who was a public fixture now turned recluse.

But one person noticed, suspected what was happening, and understood. My next door neighbour invited me over one day for a chat to reveal his battle with the illness. I was surprised and relieved to the point that I opened up as well. Here was a man whom I regarded as an oak, with a strong personality and sense of character. Yet, like me, he had private battles with a misunderstood disease. For the first time, I realized it wasn't about failure or personality profiling. For depression is no respecter of persons.

Life went on as it should and presented me a new career with new challenges. While tools for managing stress weren't obvious or provided, there were also side effects associated with my medication, an unfortunate by-product of keeping depression at bay. Through many discussions with my doctor, a new med was prescribed that solved all of the previous physical problems yet created a new one: constant drowsiness with a never-ending thirst for sleep. Like many side effects, this one was not immediately obvious or attributable to the med. It discreetly entered my life patterns and took a tremendous toll on work to the point where performance could no longer keep up with expectations.

Like many things about depression just a few short years ago, access to care and information was available but limited, especially in a rural area of the province. Some doctors prescribed with reluctance, and substitutions with more caution. Clearly, a holistic approach to depression was required to control it, rather than it controlling me.

Facing the end of another career and doubling the feeling of failure, I trudged off to a new position in Alberta. Jobs were plentiful and the pay was good. It seemed my past in Gander had prevented me from a new future and moving on appeared to be the only solution. But proper treatment available for depression was still lacking, and any decisions made under these circumstances were subject to failure. I was living in Alberta alone and 5000 kilometres from family and friends. Within five months any emotional defense I had left was completely broken down, and returning home was the only option.

My confidence shaken beyond measure, I returned to St. John's to stay with my mother, and started seeking treatment immediately. If failure had been the feeling before, complete ineptitude was the order of the day. I feared going to simple places like Costco, in the event someone from my past would be there and I'd have to explain why I returned. Stories were invented and given to people I knew. A select few knew the truth, and that dressed up to appear more palatable than it actually was.

I applied for disability only to find the process demeaning, long, and arduous at best. It left a sense of insecurity at a time of extreme vulnerability. Paying premiums all my working life should have entitled me to the very benefit deserved, but on a fateful Friday evening, my insurer called to say that I didn't meet the criteria under my policy. I was living off the graces of my mother, no income, and feeling like I had no reason to live.

I drove around the city, contemplating where I would park and take the overdose when words by my sister echoed in my mind. "If it ever gets that bad, get yourself to a hospital," she said. Thankfully, there was a shred of reason left and I presented myself at the Waterford for immediate intervention. My struggles were long from over but the healing process could at last begin.

I was referred to the START program offered by Eastern Health and began intake treatment shortly thereafter. Finally, a holistic approach was available, and included team-style intervention by a psychiatrist, psychologist, and group therapy sessions. Medications have been adjusted as necessary while cognitive-based therapy is providing new coping skills. Words cannot express my gratitude to my treating professionals.

After a six-month long ordeal, which included three appeals, a lawyer, five hours of telephone interviews, eight letters, reports from two GPs, two psychologists and two psychiatrists, my insurer granted the claim. It was clear that they and my employer had a limited understanding of depression and any criteria that would prevent working under the definitions contained in the policy. Ironically, a time ideally reserved for recovery was deeply scarred by fighting for a fundamental cause.

As I reflect on the past few years and look ahead to the next, there are stark realities which govern my life. Managing depression is attainable yet a full-time job in itself. Returning to work has still been hampered by this, and further by the lack of a re-integration program. It would appear that my current employer does not wish to accommodate my illness, and despite the façade of political correctness, most new employers may feel the same way. Yes I'm entitled to privacy, but it's only as good as society's leniency to accommodate it.

In closing, submitting these thoughts has been an exercise in confronting stigma. I do so with the belief that walls are coming down in society, but still have a ways to go. It has also been an exercise in demonstrating hope. If but one is inspired to seek help, it makes the exposure worth it. All the words of wisdom sound the same, but please know you are not alone. If you find yourself contemplating the value of your life some day, please know that you are never alone.

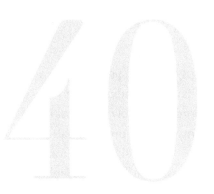

ROAD TO A GOOD LIFE

Linda Walker, Winterton, NL

So many psychiatric hospitalizations in recent years! I could hardly believe it when I checked over my records. I have always been a very organized, sometimes obsessive person in keeping records, dates, lists of medications, and so forth, so when I decided to try and put this into writing this essay I reviewed the files.

Now I know — BIPOLAR DEPRESSION!! It finally has a name, after all these years.

Bipolar is an exaggeration of your emotions, so when you get knocked down by life, it is very hard to bounce back, therein the repeated recurring incidents over the years, almost like migraines which come on suddenly and you have no control or knowledge of why or how it happened. Heredity also is a contributing factor.

I described it to people as "feeling like you were in a dark, deep pit and sinking even further down and unable to see any hope." Your thinking becomes so distorted that you see yourself as inadequate and undeserving of love and only a burden to those around you. You go through a gamut of human emotions: excess of sorrow and joy, unhappiness, impulsivity, racing thoughts and irritability.

I convinced myself on so many occasions that although I had a caring and loving husband and son, they would be better off without me and that I was only bringing them down. I justified these thoughts to the point where most of my attempts were overdoses, followed by hospitalizations. The *impaired insight and distorted thoughts* would see me blaming my husband for things he wouldn't do or cutting myself off from people to alienate myself as much as I could. This illness is so very difficult for family members to cope with as well. For years I could not understand what I was dealing with and how it affected me and others around me.

It may have begun in the late seventies (although I recall feeling depressed often as a teenager). I felt that anxiety was taking over my life; I would leave the house and walk for hours — only to have to walk back and feel like my insides were going to explode. I felt like a caged lion, pacing around the house. I had a small son and was so afraid of losing control. I had a job that I loved and was good at, but had to quit due to the inability to cope. I sought help in Montreal — a psychiatrist who really just listened, but offered no insight as to what I was dealing with. When I left Montreal, to help my anxiety she gave me two months' supply of Rivotril to which I became addicted. A hospitalization in Montreal was of no benefit whatsoever.

The move to Newfoundland (something I had wanted, but didn't realize how difficult an adjustment it would be) put an added strain on me. I was now living in a remote outport community of approximately 600 people, with virtually no immediate family or friends for support and where access to help was difficult and the stigma of mental illness is even more pronounced. The very public ambulance-to-hospital trips made me a well-known "mentally-ill person" in the community.

I would impulsively take off for days at a time, check myself into a hotel to escape, to be alone, with my husband not knowing where I was or how I was. Overdoses were done on impulse, not actual death wishes but more to stop the suffering. I would pray at night that I would die in my sleep and join my parents, who I missed terribly, or while driving, would have thoughts of just steering off the road or hoping someone would run into me. I would try to reason with God and try to convince myself that *He* would understand my suffering and need to escape.

In between all of this chaos, we were running a small convenience store where I had responsibilities (store sales, bookkeeping, and so forth), which I somehow managed to fulfill.

Early on my GP would admit me to a local hospital as a safety precaution. This in itself was stressful because none of the nursing staff in these small outport hospitals were equipped to deal with mental illness of any kind and most would run in, leave my medication and run out, afraid of what they were dealing with. One nurse even made jokes to me about not leaving a small plastic knife in my presence — to which I responded quite verbally that she obviously did not understand how difficult it was to cope with this illness. When this was not enough, admission to a psychiatric unit in St. John's was the best and most effective treatment. Finally — people were there to help me!!

Misdiagnoses were popping up everywhere through the years: depressive disorder, anxiety disorder, unipolar disorder, endogenous depression, and so forth. But it felt like no one could help me get a grip on it all.

Around 1993, I was assigned to a mental health social worker at the local hospital (part of the Eastern Health services) who, to this day, remains the one stabilizing factor in my dealing with my mental health issues. She was and is always there for me at a moment's notice and has provided the *immediate* sounding board I so need and the invaluable insight into my illness: the understanding that I had an ILLNESS that I was *not responsible for* and had to learn to cope and live with.

Just being able to talk to someone immediately about all the raw emotions I was having, the confusing ups and downs I did not understand, saved me, I'm sure, from giving up all together. I will be forever grateful for this person coming into my life at just the right time. She taught me the most valuable lesson of all over the years: to look out for yourself, be good to yourself and only YOU can make yourself happy.

There's an article I have seen on the Internet — that God sends people into your life at just the right time — either for a reason, season or a lifetime. I became determined then to get as much information as I could to understand depression — how it works and how to cope with it. There were periods when I would decide I didn't need the medications — only to fall deeper into the "pit" once again and be readmitted. Once I accepted that this was a chemical imbalance that I could not control, only then was I ready to face it head-on.

Again God sent a very gifted psychologist into my life for a few years, who through cognitive therapy and hard work on my part helped me understand how a depressive illness affects my life, and I worked hard learning how to change my thinking and deal with my negative thoughts. He was also gifted at boosting my confidence on each visit and helping me to realize I was able to process all of this and deal with it.

I could give you a list a mile long of the various medications I have been through: Ativan, Anafranil, Elavil, Prozac, Effexor, Seroquel, and others. They certainly played a part in treating the anxiety and depression. Through the one psychiatrist who finally knew what to do: it took the exact right combination of antidepressants and anxiety medication to stabilize me. Dedicated people — social worker, psychologist, psychiatric nurses, psychiatrist, as well as a course in the Day Program — were the real contributing forces in my accepting my illness and coping with it. When I worried one time what the people in the outport would think of me, my psychologist said that "*a good life is the best revenge*" — and I worked very hard to create "a good life."

It is so true what they say: that what doesn't kill you makes you stronger. I look back now five years since my last hospitalization, and depression and anxiety seem to be under control. (One is never quite sure that it won't reoccur). I maintain my medication and do not stray from the exact mix that works for me.

At times some things become overwhelming and it feels like you are slipping once again, but the episodes are shorter and the ability to cope is much better due to the education I underwent and the wonderful people who were there for me. You come out of this with a certain amount of wisdom.

I no longer worry about what others think. I live my life with the spiritual guidance of the Lord and help and love from the people who were always there for me and still are helping me along the way one day at a time. Throughout the "dark" years of my illness I still managed to find time to volunteer in the local school and in the local seniors' home and keep myself involved in life as much as I was able. If I could offer any kind of encouragement or advice to people dealing with any type of mental illness, it would be to put your illness into perspective, realize it is not your fault, seek out the professionals who can help — don't give up till you find the right one who helps you — and last of all, realize that you are not alone, that if I can come out of it a stronger and more productive person, so can you!!

A Prayer I Relied On:
Give me the strength to be who I must be, to do what I must do.
Give me the courage to stand strong against my fears,
and have the will to express my feelings and needs.
Help me to realize I have the power to change,
no matter what anyone tells me — because of you.
Give me the faith, Lord, I need to believe in you always —
even when it seems you are not there.
Amen

WHICH ROADS TO CHOOSE

Anonymous

Home, jail, group homes, foster homes. I've lived in all these places and in both Newfoundland and Ontario. I am eighteen.

My story starts when I moved to Ontario. My parents had divorced. My mom met a man over the Internet and she decided to move my brother and me to Ontario. I thought it would be good when I was on my way up there. But on the first day of school, a guy asked me if I smoked weed. I told him I had, and so at lunch time we smoked it together. Soon we were meeting before school, lunch time, and after school to smoke weed. One day my mom caught me. She and her boyfriend said they didn't mind me smoking on the weekends. But I kept it up every day. It made me feel better. I didn't care what was going on. I was in a special needs class. I felt dumb, stupid. All my friends were in regular class. I was different.

When I was thirteen or fourteen my friend's mom bought us a half case of beer each. That was my first time drinking. Soon I was doing that on a regular basis too. I smoked weed and drank every day I could. My drug use led to heavier drug use. One May 24th weekend I bought Ecstasy for my friend and me to try. It made me feel like everything was better then in life. For the whole summer we were pretty much doing that. We were popping pills like candy. Ecstasy made me feel great but when I was coming down from it my back hurt, and my jaw pained from grinding my teeth. I even chipped a couple of pieces off them. So I would drink, so I wouldn't feel so bad.

Drugs and alcohol — that's what I was doing when I started high school. School was hard for me. I didn't usually show up. I saw no point. I struggled with academics, and school was not a comfortable place. I was always being searched for drugs. Even though there was a "cop shop" in my school it didn't change what I did. I eventually just stopped going.

After Christmas I started to do coke and drank almost every day. I couldn't afford my habits, so I started stealing to finance them. I started going to drug houses with older people in their forties. We used to sell off what we had stolen in exchange for drugs. We used to do our drugs there.

Eventually I started getting watched by cops. They brought me in for questioning. They put me in a holding cell. I denied everything. They let me out. My mom came and picked me up. A week later they caught me doing something, but released me on a promise to appear in court. A week after that we did a crime and the cops chased us. I got away but then a few days after, two undercover cops arrested me. This time they brought me to another town. I waited in a holding cell to go to court. My mom didn't show up this time. They sent me to a detention centre. I was there for two weeks, got out, got in trouble, got put back! I was incarcerated in April, did detox, got out in July.

When I got out I went to Newfoundland to live with my aunt. I was clean for about two months but then I started smoking weed again and drinking. She wanted me not to do it. She wanted me to move in with my dad. I hadn't seen him in two years. When we met again, I saw that he was an alcoholic and into drugs. We did coke together. My aunt freaked out, called an ambulance. I ended up in Emergency, hooked up to monitors. I got out the next day. My aunt couldn't handle what had happened. She called the social worker and I was put into a group home.

It was easier to get charged in there. Any bad behaviour (a breach) they could call the cops. My social worker found me a foster home in Conception Bay South. A few weeks later I was drinking too much. I got glass in my finger and went to Emergency. They called the cops. I don't remember much — just waking up in a holding cell with cuts and bruises. My new foster mother told me it took five police officers to restrain me. I was sent to a detention centre.

My foster parents came to visit me. We were only allowed ten minutes. They said they'd take me back. When the ten minutes were up they had to leave. They weren't allowed to hug me or have any contact with me. That was the last time I was in custody.

After all that I went to a psychiatrist. She prescribed me medication that really helped me in school because it helped me concentrate. The school I attended, District school, really helped me. The teachers understood my anxiety and sent me for testing with my school problems.

I discovered that my learning problems came from a learning disability. I learned that a learning disability does not mean that I am stupid or dumb. I just process information differently.

I am now doing the Adult Basic Education (ABE) program at the College of the North Atlantic and I have access to the technology that puts me on an equal playing field. I know I can finish school and go on to post-secondary. I'd like to be a conservation officer and work outdoors.

If it wasn't for my foster parents, and supportive schools, instead of sitting down writing this story I would probably be in bars or behind bars.

PRESENTATION FOR PARTNERSHIP WORKSHOP

John Collins, St. John's, NL
Submitted by his mother Irene Collins

My son John Halley Collins was a very warm, loving person who accepted having the serious mental illness of schizophrenia with grace, humour, and a determined attitude to make a difference by giving presentations about the disease and his personal experiences with the many effects on his life. He was a good communicator and reached many health care professionals, police, and school children among the many groups he spoke to. He had a unique ability to do this and became an effective mental health educator.

This presentation is an early example of his work and is included here to demonstrate his ability to reach people openly and to help remove some stigma. Unfortunately his medications took their toll and caused physical deterioration in the form of overweight, diabetes, and sleep apnea, to which he succumbed on April 23, 2005, at the age of forty-two. He was a very brave person.

Irene Collins

Ten years' university training. What degree or certificate would one expect from such a lengthy time in school? A Ph.D.? A Master's degree? An M.D.?

The reality of having schizo-affective disorder, which began in high school, has led me to look upon my degree as my biggest achievement.

It is a degree in perseverance as much as it is a degree in sociology. Dealing with hospitalizations, the lethargy caused by both the disease and the treatment, along with other, more usual problems that students face, make university achievement problematic at best for [mental health] consumers.

Few things are as devastating as landing in the hospital for the first, the second, the third time, each time calling a halt to any sort of productive activity. There is something about those moments of realization that led me to believe that I had not only failed, but failed miserably and finally. It takes between six months to a year to fully recover from episodes like I have had — and these are considered to be one's prime years.

Watching my peers graduate, move on, move away and gain their independence was crushing to my self-image — but it made me more and more determined to attain an education.

I consider myself to be a very fortunate consumer. For some reason, unknown to me, I am usually very well between episodes, allowing me to reach some of my goals, though not on the timetable I would choose.

A key factor in completing a degree was my family's support. Without the emotional, intellectual and financial help I received from my family it would likely have taken me twice the time to have done half as much. I realize that not all consumers have this resource.

I am also thankful to those members of the faculty and administration of Memorial University for their understanding and accommodation to my needs as a student with mental illness.

I don't feel quite the same way about my experience in high school. I suffered two mind-numbing, gut-wrenching depressions during those years. As with most students suffering mental illness in high school, the embarrassment, shame and guilt, accompanied by confusion as to what was happening, led to isolation, misery, and to lower grades. No one in my school reached out to me — not one teacher or student. But what could I have expected? There was no place for discussing such problems, much less solving them.

The only memory I have of any teacher noticing my dilemma was when I received a poor mark on a math test. There was a note on it saying, "When are you going to take this course seriously?" And that was it. High school was for me a bleak, empty place. I suppose that my teachers assumed that I was a quiet person by nature, uninterested in school or socializing.

It was encouraging and refreshing to attend the CMHA/Lawton's Youth Speak-Off last December and hear that high school students and teachers are now talking about and dealing with mental health issues. Initiatives like these are crucial to opening up the eyes of both students and teachers.

At this time I'd like to relate a story coming out of my work experience which will underscore the need for education and openness about mental illness.

For two summers in my early twenties, I worked with a social service agency and received excellent feedback on my performance. In the fall of the second year I was offered, and accepted, a new, temporary assignment from the director of that agency. The problem was that I was slipping into a manic episode. My behaviour was becoming more and more unusual: I was becoming more talkative, more intolerant of others' points of view, and behaving more inappropriately.

The new work situation I was entering into only served to heighten the mania. I have no question in my mind now that I needed to be off work at that time — I could not do the job properly. However, while experiencing the mania, I was convinced that I was extraordinarily well. Except for one co-worker, no one at the office even for a moment recognized the mania for what it was. And, therefore, no one suggested sick leave, which would have been suggested for any other illness.

There were five social workers including the manager working in the same office as myself; the manager described me naively to a co-worker, making a moral judgement on my behaviour. And that was in response to my co-worker suggesting I might have a mental health illness.

This co-worker had known me for the two previous summers and could therefore see the drastic change in my behaviour. However, to everyone else with whom I was working, I had some sort of character defect. No one seemed to question how I had gone from excellent work to substandard work or why my previous co-workers had found me competent.

I was subsequently given one week's notice that I was fired. Recollection of this period of my life still causes me to feel angry. However, I bring this up not to blame but to point out that even in what might be considered an aware and supportive environment — an office full of social workers — ignorance about mental health abounds.

Currently, I work three days per week in a family business. Again, I feel I am fortunate to have my family's support and the opportunity to take time off when my health is not so good. I know three other consumers who work for their families and it seems for some to be a way around the problem of stigma and employment barriers. Most consumers do not have this opportunity.

All this having been said, I would like to put forth two suggestions. First, social workers, during their training, should be required to complete compulsory work terms in a mental health setting. I say this because mental illness and mental health problems are so common among people who use social work services.

The second is that high schools should have time set apart from health education to include education about the realities of mental illness and mental health hygiene.

And the fact remains that education for employers and teachers, as well as supports for those with mental illness and mental health problems, remains of critical importance.

A JOURNEY TO HELL

Clayton Hunt, Harbour Breton, NL

"You've been in Hell!"

"Yes, I've been there, my friend, and I can tell you that it's not a pretty place. Believe me, you don't want to go there."

"I thought you had to die to go to Hell. And that you had to have been really evil."

"Oh, no, not at all. You don't have to be dead to get to this Hell, and you don't have to be evil at all. Anyone can go to this Hell."

"I haven't heard many people talk about this. I suppose you're the only one who has been in this Hell."

"Oh, no no. Thousands, millions have been in this Hell. Millions of people are probably there this very day."

"How long were you in this Hell?"

"At the time it seemed like an eternity. Looking back now it was only a month for me. Some people are there much longer than that. Some are there for years and years."

"I thought you didn't get out of Hell once you got there."

"I was one of the lucky ones, I guess. It's a place you don't think you will ever leave but with professional help and support from family and friends many people get out to lead normal lives again."

"So, everyone gets out of this Hell?"

"No, unfortunately some people never get out. They never get a chance to leave as they end their own lives."

"Did you try to commit suicide, to take your own life?"

"Yes."

"Why? It amazes me that a person would try to do that as life is a precious thing and we only get a little time on the planet."

"Well, people all over the world do it. Most people do it alone but some people do it in groups or cults."

"You're talking about depression right?"

"Yes, severe depression, the deepest, darkest, ugliest kind where you feel that terrible sinking feeling in your stomach like it's going to be sucked out through your back and nothing in your life will ever be the same again."

"This Hell you refer to is on Earth then?"

"Yes."

"By the way, what causes depression?"

"A professional told me that a major cause is a traumatic change in your life, like the death of a loved one or retirement, which causes a chemical imbalance in the brain."

"In your case?"

"In my case it was retirement."

"Tell me your story."

"I'm not sure if I can explain what happened now, if I can make sense of it or if there is any sense to it. Are you sure you really want to hear about this?"

"Yes."

First of all I want to make it perfectly clear that what happened to me was my own fault. No other person is remotely responsible for what transpired in my life in the fall of 2002.

I retired from the teaching profession in Newfoundland in June 2002 after twenty-eight years in the profession. I bought back two university years as work service years so I could retire two years earlier than I normally would have.

I had attended a retirement seminar in Grand Falls-Windsor where the Newfoundland and Labrador Teachers' Association officials told us to be prepared for retirement — to have something to do after you left teaching, mainly to keep your mind occupied.

Of course, I didn't believe them. I thought I could pass my days by reading, watching television, surfing the Internet and by just lounging around the house.

I was okay during the summer of 2002 and in September we went to visit our daughter in Halifax. I can remember my daughter asking me if I was going to be okay and I said, Sure, I'll be fine.

It wasn't too long after we got back from Halifax that I started to feel different about some aspects of my life. I didn't realize it at the time, but I was starting to become depressed.

I was feeling guilty about retiring early and I came to believe that I had let my wife and family down. In all my life I had never worried about money before, but now I got to believing that my wife and I would not be able to make it financially. My wife told me I was being foolish but the feeling persisted.

I got to thinking, for example, that we would not be able to keep up with the light bills, and the power people would cut the electricity to our house or that we would lose our phone and cable television.

I would be home most days alone as my wife was working, and I would literally beat myself up thinking about these things and all the not-so-bright things I had done in my life. I got to feeling worthless and very stupid. I couldn't sleep and I lost weight like you wouldn't believe.

The weight literally melted away as I went back to 175 pounds after battling weight around the 200-pound mark for many years. It was like food was doing me no good at all.

It got to the point where I lost all interest in the little things that make life enjoyable. I lost interest in reading (and I'm an avid reader), watching sports such as American football, which I really look forward to each fall, television, movies, and music.

Just getting out of bed in the morning was like a Herculean task. I had to work up the courage to shave or to have a shower as I didn't care about my appearance at all. I didn't want to be out in crowds and the nighttime seemed like my only friend.

Slowly, ever so slowly, but ever so surely, it dawned on me that if I couldn't enjoy those things in life, then what was the point of it all? This feeling, combined with the terrible guilt and the inactivity, led me to become suicidal. It was like I had committed the most terrible crime in letting my family down. I was the judge and the jury and the only sentence was death.

I was going through a very rough time and so was my wife. I was very naïve as I thought I could be depressed and that she could go on with her life. Of course, it wasn't like that.

Because I couldn't sleep and was up throughout the night, my wife wasn't getting her proper rest. There were days when she went to work without a good night's sleep and her worrying about me was affecting her work to some degree. Depression not only affects the victim but the entire family as well. It was only the wife and me at home now and she was going through her personal Hell as well.

In the meantime I had gone to seek professional help and the doctor knew right away I was depressed. I was on certain medications which seemed to be working and maybe I should have given the medication more time. The doctor too wanted me to see a nurse physiatrist. I did see this particular nurse after, and I realize now that I should have seen her when the doctor actually wanted me to.

I can remember December 3 of that year. That night I was sort of on a high as I was listening to some music on my computer before going to bed. However, the next morning when I woke I could feel that sinking feeling again and I had to struggle to get out of bed. I honestly felt that I would try and end my life that day.

Speaking about ending my life, I had been suicidal for a fairly long time, at least for two months or so. I had thought about committing suicide and if I had had access to a suicide pill I sincerely think I wouldn't be here today. I don't have a gun, although I doubt I would have used one to kill myself anyway.

At night in bed I would pray to God, asking Him to take my life as I didn't want to face another day. At Lions meetings or with friends I would ask myself, "Who else is suicidal here?" I don't know if there are degrees of being suicidal, but I had to be as suicidal as you can get.

On December 4, 2002, I realized that, while I didn't have one suicide pill, I could take an overdose of pills to kill myself. My wife had some pills hidden in the house but I found them.

That afternoon a friend of mine and I had agreed to go for a walk but I just didn't have the courage or the energy to go. When he phoned and asked me why I didn't show up, I said I couldn't get the car started.

That afternoon, around 3:30 or 4, I took the pills and drank some rum I had in the house. I can't remember how many pills I took — it was quite a few. After taking the pills I went in the room and lay down on the bed to die. My wife came home around 5 and woke me with her knocking, as I had locked the door.

I got up and tried to pretend nothing had happened. However, it didn't take my wife too long to figure out something was terribly wrong with me, and she figured out what I did pretty quickly.

She got our next door neighbours to come in and they took me to the hospital. The doctor on call that night gave me an antidote to the pills I had taken and they got me up to Grand Falls-Windsor where I spent the next three weeks in the intensive care unit and in the psychiatric ward.

My treatment at Grand Falls-Windsor was pretty good, I guess. I wish the physiatrists there had more time for me, but I guess there were so many people to see they couldn't spend all day with me. While all the staff at the hospital were good, there were two nurses, one male and one female, who treated me with great kindness and helped me get back on my feet.

My wife, who had gone through a terrible time with me during my depression, was there for me at the hospital as was my extended family and friends. One of my friends sent me in four bottles of Pepsi and I appreciated that more than receiving cash at the time.

I had a niece who was living in Grand Falls-Windsor at the time who, although she didn't know me that well, was really good to me.

I remember one night she brought me up some fried salmon fillets, and Jesus, were they ever good. She may think I've forgotten the kindness she showed me but I haven't. I'll never forget it and I hope I can repay the favour some day.

I was at the hospital until December 22 when officials allowed me to return home for Christmas. The funny thing is I wasn't sure if I really wanted to come home at the time. My son and wife were there to take me home, but it seemed so safe there and I wasn't sure if I wanted to face the world again.

I was home for the Christmas season and it wasn't long before life started getting back to its usual routine. That Christmas, friends visited and several couples came to the house to play cards one night. For New Year's Eve we went to a friend's house to play cards.

After Christmas I went back to the Lions Club. A friend there who had gone through a difficult time himself encouraged me to come back to the club and I was glad I did shortly after, although it took a while to get back to being comfortable around people.

I think it was in January of 2003 when I received a phone call one night from the principal of St. Joseph's School asking me to come back to be the secretary of the school council as I had been secretary for several years. I remember walking into the school and actually entering the library where the meeting was being held. Everyone else was there, and to talk in that room was a major task. It seemed like I couldn't' do it but I did and things were fine after.

My life slowly returned to its normal routine. I saw a nurse physiatrist for a few months and I'm still on certain medications to this day. I'd like to wean off the pills but my wife doesn't want me to try it now. Maybe I can later on.

I'm doing pretty well now. I've done some substitute teaching, and in November 2004 when the Fisheries Products International fish plant in Harbour Breton closed, the editor of our local Transcontinental weekly newspaper called me to ask me to do some writing for her as I had worked with the paper before.

Today I still do some freelance writing for the paper, a task I really love to do. Just to get out and meet people, the feeling of being a part of the workforce, of contributing to society, well, to me that's better than all the medication in the world.

They say things happen for a reason. I don't know about these things. I've met some wonderful people since my depressions, two editors in particular and especially a little girl in Gaultois who I may have never got to know so well if I had not retired early.

We have a grandson in Halifax now who is the light of my life and who gives me a new reason to go on with life. In recent years I've never felt depressed like I did in 2002. I hope I never do again but you don't know about these things.

Why did I try to kill myself? I'm not sure if I can give you an exact answer. I was feeling guilty for retiring early and for what I thought was letting my wife down. I sincerely believed that I deserved death for what I did. I know that may sound strange but I was convinced of that then and nothing could change my mind.

I try to make sense of it all today but it's hard to do. Some people say that suicide is a permanent solution to a temporary problem, and I guess that's true. Maybe suicide is the cowardly way out. I didn't think we could make it financially and maybe suicide was a way out.

"Your story was very interesting but what's the point? Why did you want to let people know about this? Why bring up these painful memories again?"

"Because depression can happen to anyone at any time. It can catch you off guard and sneak up on you so fast you don't even know it's happening until it's too late. But no matter how depressed you get, you can seek help and you can recover with that help from professionals, family, and friends.

"I know the dark may seem like it will never end and you think your life will never be the same. Just don't forget that the greatest gift of all is another day, a day that can change your life for the better, and that you can be well again."

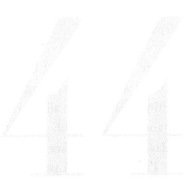

COMING BACK

Stephen Gale, Kelowna, BC

The doors onto and off of the ward were always locked. The windows were bulletproof thick and not of the opening variety. I used to dream of wwii-esque escapes from the stalag — or vanishing down the castle wall on a rope of tied together bedsheets . . . but that was the madness. I was four floors up in a psychiatric hospital in Newfoundland. I had signed myself in, but two or three doctors had subsequently committed me . . . so I was in for some kind of long haul.

When I went in, they had no idea what was on the go with me. Drug-related psychosis? Schizo-affective such and such? Hypomania? They didn't know. They started in with the usual (for 1995) round of anti-psychotics for psychosis, horse tranquilizers for sleep . . . and all the rest. The grocer's list of drugs I was on for the month and a half I was inside would be as long as your arm. I wasn't sleeping. I didn't need to eat too much. I felt like I could walk a twenty-mile day on water and adrenaline. I rambled incoherently to everyone but myself (and, of course, some of the other likewise gifted patients making up my ward). Thoughts and the thought process seemed to be pregnant with a nascent possibility. And that proliferated endlessly . . . topic reeled into topic which turned into something else and it was all fascinating.

Truth was, I could barely stay on one topic for more than a

minute. I had a beard I hadn't trimmed in six months. I was flat broke. I stank. Everything was possible. But that's not why I'm writing this today, to all who care to listen. I'm not going to tell you all 2000 words' worth of manic recollection and impatience with today's psychiatric care and method.

I'm going to tell you, in 500 words or less, how I managed to come back. I had a family that cared. Nothing would have happened without them. I, quite literally, owe them my life twice over at least. Without the love of my father and mother and brother, I would be nowhere. Emotion from people you love is probably the most important aspect of any recovery.

I had friends who cared. Emotion from them was just as important as that from family.

Exercise. One of the single most important aspects of any recovery is possible by yourself. No shrink ever told me this. And I mean vibrant, ongoing physical exercise. I go for long walks hours away from wherever, endlessly — whenever I can. Backpack, bottle of water, sandwich, and go. We were not meant to sit on couches forever and a day. Ride a bike. Have sex. Go for a jog. Don't put all your faith in the pills. They help. They may help you build a cornerstone from which to drag yourself from the mire . . . if you're lucky . . . the side effects won't be so bad. Psychiatric theory these days is one of the best answers we have at the moment. Most in the system know it's not the right one, however. But it's the best we have right now. Good mental health doesn't come in a bottle . . . however much big pharma would love you to think so. So many of the mentally ill have just forgotten about the beauty of their own lives and end up getting medicated at a crossroads where they should have actually just turned left.

Speech. Talk to people. Other folks who have dragged themselves through these hells know, and talking to them makes the nightmare easier to put into some kind of context. A context of the rest of your life. Don't watch too much TV.

Stigma. Wel-l-l-l-l . . . always remember that the stigma associated with any given subject is directly related to how much it is *mis*-understood. Don't try to reinvent the wheel talking to folks about your illness. Lots of people can't, or do not want to, understand madness. It terrifies them. Good mental health is an individual thing. It takes your whole life to learn your individual variety, and learn it well. Take with a healthy grain of salt the advice of psychiatrists. Trust your intuition.

Rest. Slow down. Turn off the rapidly cycling engines. Remember always that paranoia is just the frenetic version of self-doubt.

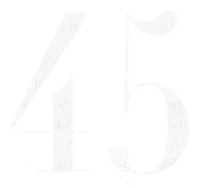

SPARK

Kim Wilton, St. John's, NL

It is sometimes hard for me to tell where I begin and my illness ends. My life has been so intimately entwined with my mental illness, it is hard for me to remember my life without it or who I am without it. I have suffered from depression and anxiety since I was a young teenager.

When you suffer from depression you become enclosed within yourself, and there is no escape. Depression descends upon you like a fog. You cannot see right in front of you and all colours fade away. It is as if your brain revolts against your body, and all your senses become muted. You become paralyzed, unable to leave your bed, let alone your house, for days and weeks on end.

Even though mental illness has been such a large part of my life, I rarely tell people that I suffer from one, even some of my closest friends do not know about it. When you tell someone that you suffer from a mental illness, you can see yourself changing right before their eyes. A divide opens up between them and you, creating a line few dare cross. There are different reactions: some people are unfailingly sympathetic and understanding, relating stories of their own struggles or stories about people they know who are "just like that" or who "had that too." While others view you either as a self-absorbed narcissist or as weak and delicate — flawed. But the reaction of most people is that, sadly, they just don't know how to act around you, they tiptoe around you, sugar-coating the world for you, afraid if they say or do the wrong thing you'll break into a million pieces in front of them.

Even though mental illness is so prevalent in our society, it is still a mark, a label, a stigma. My own experience has led me to treat my illness as a secret that I keep carefully hidden. I have become an expert at crafting elaborate stories to cover my illness, and I have developed an arsenal of lies for different situations: the "I can't go out tonight because I'm studying" excuse for when my anxiety is so high I cannot bear the thought of leaving my house, or the "I've been having terrible migraines" excuse to explain my absence from school when I cannot leave my bed for days, or even weeks, on end.

Mental illnesses are, above all, very lonely diseases. There are no get-well cards, flowers or visitors, only silence. Time and time again, I have wished that I suffered from a "real" disease, a disease where I would say "I'm sick" without the stigma that inevitably follows with a mental illness. Even the closest and most intimate relationships become twisted and tried under the strain of a mental illness. While some close friends may initially be supportive and understanding, even these friendships tend to crumble under the burden.

Yet, for all the heartache and misery that my mental illness has caused me, it has also taught me some valuable lessons. Your true friends are revealed, the people who will stick with you through anything. It has also taught me compassion, empathy and has even given me strength. If you've lived through a mental illness you can live through anything.

LIVING WITH BIPOLAR DISORDER

Janet Bartlett, Conception Harbour, NL

If someone had asked me twenty-five years ago to share my experiences with mental health, I would likely not have known how to respond. Today, I could write a novel, perhaps a series, and would still not adequately represent what it means for my sister, what it means to me or to my family. In any event, I decided to include a submission to the call for essays in a feeble attempt to be a voice for my sister, who lives each day of her life with bipolar disorder as an illness — as a label. Labels can be double-edged; they can be helpful medically when they lead to speedy diagnosis, treatment and recovery, but they can also be detrimental to the person who cannot function outside the boundaries placed upon them by that label in society. I do not pretend to imagine my sister's struggles, and so this piece is perhaps more reflective of my perspective on her mental health challenges and successes.

Bipolar disorder, as many other mental health "disorders," is characterized by recurring patterns of wellness and illness. Behaviours associated with the illness, such as mania or depression, create stigma which is very difficult to overcome. The stigma speaks to society's inability to comprehend or accept difference and is perhaps driven by fear. It also speaks to discrimination directed toward those living with mental health issues because they exist outside what is considered acceptable and "normal" by societal standards.

This does not mean to imply that characteristics of the disorder do not require treatment, but rather that a more complex understanding of how it impacts the individual and their family is needed.

People living with bipolar disorder, because of the chronic nature of the disorder, can experience many challenges such as increased unemployment and dependency on others for assistance, particularly social assistance programs. This factor alone contributes to many aspects of stigma. People living with mental health issues are often viewed as not adequately contributing to society and as a drain on social or health care resources. In addition, certain aspects of behaviour associated with the disorder do little to solicit sympathy or compassion from others who lack any real understanding of mental health disorders.

There is a belief in our individualistic society that reward comes to those who work hard and those who are emotionally and physically strong. Mental illness by contrast is viewed as a weakness, a deficiency, a disability, a burden to society. If mental illness has become a burden to society, it is because society has constructed it as such by its refusal to see individuals living with mental illness as people with the same needs, wants, and desires and basic human rights. It is society's reluctance to change its perspectives and current structures designed to "manage" people living with mental illness that has created our current, inadequate, mental health care system.

In this province, tertiary institutions with acute and long-term care facilities are still the predominant approach to treatment and care for people like my sister. This presents many challenges for families like ours since services are generally located in urban centres and focus mainly on crisis intervention and treatment as opposed to prevention or early intervention which could prevent or reduce recurrences of the disorder.

In the past, appropriate and adequate community supports in terms of continuity of care were limited to assessment prior to hospital discharge and follow-up with a family physician and/or psychiatrist. In the past five years, however, this particular aspect of care has been addressed with the introduction of a new mental health act involving the hiring of mental health liaison nurses to follow up patients after discharge from hospital. Of course the limitation of this program is that it excludes people who have not been admitted to hospital but may be unwell in the community and not receiving care. Before this act was introduced, however, there were few attempts to address issues that do not pertain directly to the illness but which are often a by-product, such as level of education, employment, income, and how these factors intersect with the illness to produce a specific lifestyle.

In addition, considering that my sister lives in St. John's and still has limited access to a more holistic approach to her situation and overall well-being, I wonder how people and families living in rural areas cope where services are further limited or nonexistent. Many people living with mental health issues function no differently in society than the majority, but there are just as many who face considerable challenges due to specific characteristics of their disorder and the limited options available to them.

While there exist some wonderful voluntary and government-funded organizations that provide support for individuals and families, it is often the stigma and the need to "forget" a relapse which may result in a person or family choosing not to avail of these particular support services. In addition, poverty, which often goes hand-in-hand with mental illness (and is highly reflective of systemic problems in society), may limit outings potentially deemed as a lower priority due to issues of transportation.

Prior to the new Mental Health Act, without supportive family members, a person living with bipolar disorder could live in isolation with periodic admissions to hospital, where care was limited to the hospital stay and individuals were released into a community with inadequate or nonexistent community supports. At least now we have mental health liaison nurses who can overcome the gap between hospital discharge and integration into the community. If we could take this one step further, such that people requiring assistance or care had immediate access to intermediary health care professionals without admission to hospital, we may be able to prevent and/or reduce hospital admissions or at the very least shorten a hospital stay. The end result of such an approach? Individuals could remain well for longer periods of time with less frequent relapses of shorter duration and fewer hospital admissions. Seems like a strategy which should be attainable, beneficial to individuals and families, cost effective, and worth the effort.

So we must ask ourselves why it is that mental health is such a low priority to our governments, our health care system, and society, and why people living with mental health disorders are considered "orphans" of Canada's health care system. Is stigma the culprit here as well? If so, what can we do to change it? I can only offer my perspective as a family member — historically excluded from my sister's care yet morally responsible for her well-being — and ask that society afford her the same dignity, respect, and compassion they would were she diagnosed with cancer rather than a mental health disorder. She deserves no less respect or admiration for her struggles, her triumphs, her losses — and she certainly has mine. I cannot begin to understand what it is like to live her life amidst so much discrimination and intolerance of difference in society. I can only speak to my experiences of her illness and the loss I feel each time she has a relapse — loss for the sister I know and love, loss of the relationship we have when she is well, and loss and frustration resulting from exclusion of her care and societal attitudes toward mental illness. So, I continue to fight and advocate for her and for all those living with mental health issues who have been silenced through societal disregard, indifference, isolation, and marginalization.

I would like this message to also serve as a reminder that we must all advocate for mental health since it is crucial to us all. We do not know how or when any of us might be impacted by that which we take for granted — our mental health.

It will be a long road to recovery for society, and for those affected, but we must begin somewhere. Education is a critical piece of this puzzle, in particular, educating the public to deconstruct popular notions and attitudes toward issues of mental health. Currently, the media, which perpetuates stereotypes of mental illness, is a prominent source of education for the general public, and this must change. Capitalizing on the suffering of individuals seems to be the status quo for ratings, with a total disregard of how that contributes to the global stigma of mental illness. In addition, we must also educate our mental health professionals to treat people not as isolated entities or disorders but rather as members of a family and of a community invested in their well-being.

And so, we must begin to deconstruct societal contributions and causes of the stigma and burden surrounding mental health issues and the families impacted. Only then can we fight for change to our health care system and health care policies for improved care, which considers not only the rights of the individuals affected but also the family who is impacted by decisions surrounding their care, and ensure adequate community and societal supports are available so they have the same opportunities to contribute and participate in society.

VENTURING FROM THE
MIASMA OF MIRTHLESSNESS

Gus Russell, St. John's, NL

My name is Gus and I am a mental health consumer. This essay explores the symptoms of my illness, provides access to a distraught mind and manifests the hope, resilience and stoicism involved in facing a deluge of delusions, paranoia, bizarre thoughts and profound depression.

Notwithstanding the fact that I do not condone the restrictions of a psychiatric label, I suffer from an affliction called schizo-affective (bipolar sub-group) disorder. It is sufficient to say that my mood is affected — from high to low. As well, my thoughts, even though there is a slight degree of rationality, penetratingly alter my concept of reality. These thoughts are considered to be bizarre. Delusions play a part, and the rest of this essay formats the struggle of two opposing forces in my self — in my mind. Such neurotransmitters as serotonin and dopamine are instrumental in determining the intensity of the depression and/or the paranoid and bizarre thoughts. However, I rule out the scientific methods of viewing the illness and concentrate on the individual and the social. I proceed with more self-piloted mental health issues — stigma, hope during the bleakest moments, the boot-strap efforts of the struggle and how these factors affect a reality that has been grotesque and frightening for too long.

Depression profoundly affects me even when I am not considered to be ill. A morbid sense of a non-purpose existence over-clouds my thoughts at the best of times, and I have to remind myself that this is "as good as it gets." In order not to succumb to these feelings, I indulge in music and books, and convince the voice in my head that he is not going to win. On several occasions, the voice has dictated me to attempt suicide, but luckily I did not.

Every thought I have is commented upon by the voice, and when the serotonin rears its ugly head, my thoughts and the voice replying to them are all depressive. For instance, I could bemoan my poverty, to which the voice would reciprocate with a reminder that I go downhill because I deserve to. Unrelentingly, the voice bolsters the depression by reinforcing the first negative thought.

The actual struggle between these two forces, the hallucinogenic and the real, is, you must admit, the accumulation of morbidity and a Catch-22 resolution. However, I realize what is occurring in my psyche, and with a determined effort and cognitive psychology, I may not be able to eliminate the voice, but I can view the situation for what it is — the real against the unreal. I compartmentalize the brain into segments and unveil the voice as the part of my mind that I push to the one side, even when I am engrossed in speaking or thinking rationally.

With these thoughts in the back of my head, I set up boundaries and relegate the voice to the status of "a burr under the saddle" of rationalization. These boundaries allow me to rise above the level of the voice. This process decreases the grip of depression upon what I would call my outer mind, and alleviates the struggle to the point where medication can work its function. However, medication cannot completely dispel the voice. Notwithstanding the value of mood stabilizers and antidepressive agents, the final culmination must be realized by the total weight of will and determination. Medication can only allay, not eliminate. Resilience and hope can only be realized after this mode of thinking completely allows a denouement of the struggle that this tries to detail. God! That means I am partway there. An increase of complementing medication and I will jump over the moon.

Paranoia and its contingent anxiety attacks create a vicious cycle. If you stand back from your mind and watch its circular paranoid progressions, you can see how ridiculously the reasoning (yes, it seems like reasoning at the time) beacons a mind that is vulnerable to a chemical change reaction. Such paranoid and bizarre thoughts as thinking you are Christ or a famous writer can be justified in a befuddled mind as having a natural foundation of proof. It is almost as if everything becomes clear, and you should shout, "Eureka."

Mania (Is the going up worth the coming down?) consists of feelings of exhilaration, expanded ego, heightened self-esteem and even omnipotence. This state of mind can be dangerous to yourself or to others. People have murdered under its influence, and the deluded manic mind can give feelings of being indestructible. Hence, you will become foolhardy to the dangers inherent in human activity. Your logic may seem elaborate, and your skills of persuasion are intense. Although you may seem to be more intelligent when you are experiencing mania, I feel that it is more like the concept of the drunken wise man. With inhibition gone and flight of ideas clearly evident, the manic person may appear more intelligent, but his lucidity won't hold up to professional scrutiny.

Once, when I was manic, I had the delusion that I was a great poet — I do write poetry — and had been made the poet laureate of Harvard University. I sat down in the rags of my misconceptions and wrote a letter to Harvard's president, telling him that his university was not fit to have someone as great a poet as me. When I "came down" I realized the humour inherent in all this.

The greatest side-effect of such exhilaration is that you will "crash" — become very depressed, often suicidally depressed. Mania may make a person feel good about himself, but the hidden doubts and the basic insecurities of the mentally ill will come to the front when the buzz has worn off.

Bizarre thoughts and paranoid delusions are the order of the day for a schizo-affective. My most intense and lingering delusion was that I was a rat. Over the years, this feeling reinforced itself, until it almost gained the irreversibility of a fixed delusion. It commenced when I was a child and developed thereafter. In my only encounter with a rat, I stared down the feral creature — he looking out of the corner of one eye. It now becomes evident — an Olanzapine realization — that we exchanged the soul of one for the other. Unmistakenly, the feeling remained with me up until today, and even though I can now counter this bizarre thought with a sprinkling of reality, I still have residual symptoms, such as not using a spoon that has a rat-tailed handle or spying the word rat ten lines before I reach it, when I am reading. It could be the word erratic, but I usually pin-point it long before reaching it. During one psychotic episode, this delusion progressed (or regressed) to the point where all the patients and staff reminded me of rats. Deep down, of course, I could realize that this was an extension of my thinking that I was a rat. Despite the remaining reminders, I can put these thoughts on the back burner, and I can function, somewhat.

Another bizarre thought scheme, which I have experienced, is thinking that my thoughts are being read. Even when I am alone, I have that feeling, and when there are others nearby, I feel that passersby know what I am thinking, and I hear their responses. Of course, I recognize such a delusion as part of my illness, but nevertheless, I feel great anguish and discomfort, due to these alterations of reality. With the voice, which I have described earlier, working vigorously to defeat my state of mind, and now to have both levels of thinking scrutinized, befuddled and responded to, my "reality equilibrium" must be intense, in order to survive mentally. It is indeed a Catch-22. Of course, such a probability that this is actually happening is remote. However, you have to concede that it is possible — anything is possible — and whose reality are we going to follow?

The occupants of the neighbouring apartment notice my every move. They know when I come and go, and what I am doing when I am home. Since there is no hole in the shared wall and since I make very little noise, the only way that they can accurately comment on my waylaid activities is by reading my mind. As I already reported, this is impossible, and thus I plead paranoia, but not insanity. My mind is as acute as ever, and the mood — thanks to the stabilizing drugs — borders on normalcy. When the Great Judge for Mental Activities calls for my plea, I can safely say that the nosy neighbours made me this way. You could say they are guilty of break and entry — the invasion of the privacy of my mind.

It is very possible that I am not paranoid at all, because they are closeted all day long and rarely venture into the miasma of life outside their realm of occupancy. But to read my mind? All this proves is that I am slightly off-centre. Do you remember the term residual symptoms, which I previously mentioned? Maybe I am just sweeping up the residue. However, what excuse do they have for their nosiness?

I contend that I go into too much detail about my travail in the pits of the schizo-affective disorder, and now turn my hand to write of the glittered sojourn back to the land of the living, and the dying. With resolution, I take upon myself the fight against my illness, the continuation of hope to somehow overcome my affliction, the resilience of one with chronic mental illness, who must avail of the briefest moments, and an element of recovery. Although this recovery abates at times, the resilience brings back a far more insightful person. We, the mentally ill, must push on, but we must not be pushed around. Stigma is not to be taken with a grain of salt. The sores of this factor in the lives of the mentally ill cannot allow such a brash brandishing of extreme torture to their wounds. However, I intend to give personal, as well as societal, examples of this maltreatment. A self-fulfilling prophesy is that the mentally afflicted are losers, therefore they are inferior. Many times in the past, I have been viewed as a loser, just because I was physically and mentally ill with severe depression — to wit, I was immobilized in both directions. To them, I was viewed as having a deficiency of manhood — I couldn't face life. My view of myself deteriorated, and the incoming communication only reinforced this vacuity.

I always wanted to enter politics, but now, due to the fact that I had 50+ shock treatments, my chances of living that down would be smeared all over the media genres. Such discrimination against those who have a mental illness runs amok, and we have very little opportunity to "make something of ourselves." Society has limited our output into its machinations, just because we are a minority, and "you never know what they might do." The prophesy of acceptance that is in vogue today — everybody who is someone is bipolar — is merely a pat on society's head for being such a nice entity to "poor Johnny" and we are limited even more by condescension than we are by fear.

Despite the stigma, despite the years of hospitalization, with advent of atypical anti-psychotic drugs I have wondrously regained a footing in the outside world, and with my attitude of stoicism and cognitive banishment of the "voice" I have at least to some degree conquered my illness. The illness still exists, but I have pushed the intruding thoughts to the side. Now it is but a throbbing back pain, and the rational sphere of my brain spearheads a strengthening resolve to go forward. Of course there will always be minor loopholes, and I may flounder temporarily. But my resilience is unabatedly cognizant of possible roadblocks and makes me a stoic in the face of relapses. I may have once been a rat, but I now smell the traps along my venture. No longer is it a venture of mirthlessness, but the receding symptoms are themselves the attributes of wellness.

Now, I work as a researcher/writer for an archives and museum, after completing more than eight years of university. My resolve to attain higher education was not stifled by my illness, and luckily my illness did not affect my intellect. Have I recovered? Perhaps it is that I have discovered rather than recovered, and I have found a way to accommodate my illness into the network of functioning in a world that may not be a rose garden, but rather a plot of land of my own.

What will my future entail? At least I will have enough sanity to embrace it. Life is but a brief sojourn and we must make the best of it, whether or not a commenting voice or a distorted thought lingers on the fringes. In this essay I have disclosed many aspects of my distortions of an evasive reality, but most of all I have disclosed my humanness.

MENTAL ILLNESS AND
THE CRIMINAL JUSTICE SYSTEM

Ron Fitzpatrick, St. John's, NL

As a community chaplain employed by a not-for-profit organization known as Turnings, I have worked with many people afflicted with one or more forms of mental illness. All too often I have watched while many of these individuals fell through the cracks in our health care system only to find themselves smack-dab in the middle of the criminal justice system. Some of these people have addictions problems and are living a life filled with pain and despair.

All the things that individuals without mental illness take for granted are a monumental task for most of them: taking a bus, shopping for food and other necessities, doing laundry, proper hygiene, managing an apartment, cooking, managing their finances, and the list goes on. There is also a portion of the criminal element in our province who physically, mentally and sexually abuse many of our province's mentally ill. It is a common occurrence for criminals to enter the home or apartment of a mentally ill person and steal their belongings and warn them not to call the police or they will come back and severely harm them.

The mentally ill people we have worked with at Turnings all had or have criminal records. In some cases stealing to acquire drugs or alcohol was the cause for some to enter prison. Sometimes individuals with mental illness associate with or have a relationship with people who are mentally ill like themselves or even more severely challenged, and in almost all cases this relationship ends up with one or both individuals serving prison time. When a mentally ill person goes to prison he or she does extremely hard time. Too often they are abused by other inmates. Also, they may have some or all of their medications withheld from them if the medical personnel at the prison feel that this is appropriate. When this happens the individual most often gets totally out of sorts and suffers deep depression and acute anxiety, which in turn causes the person to lash out at other inmates or staff, and the result is that the individual is taken to solitary confinement which could even cause them to commit suicide. It has been our experience that too many mentally ill individuals leave provincial prisons in very bad physical and mental health simply because they don't fit in and their mental illness prohibits them from following normal rules and regulations. This is further compounded by the fact that provincial prisons are not equipped to properly and safely house and control people with mental illnesses.

At Turnings we believe it is morally and ethically wrong to sentence a mentally ill human being to serve time in any of our provincial prisons. These people need to be cared for at a hospital or facility such as the forensic unit at the Waterford Hospital in St. John's. We realize that there is presently limited space at this unit; however, the powers that be must act responsibly and extend and expand this unit to handle the ever-growing case load. If our health care system is going to encourage mentally ill individuals to live outside the hospital on their own, they must make sure they receive the resources they require to remain healthy and safe within our communities. If caregivers and respite workers are needed, they must be supplied. Safe and affordable lodging must be provided and people must have access on a regular basis to their own personal doctor and social worker and any other service that may be required to make sure that they don't ever again fall through the cracks in the health care system.

Too many individuals with mental health issues are forced to live on social assistance; as a result they find themselves living in lodgings that are so vile words can't properly describe the deplorable conditions forced upon them. They live out of soup kitchens and food banks and most of their clothing is second-hand. Many of these people can truly be looked upon as lost souls. What really upsets us at Turnings is the fact that when any of these mentally ill individuals get caught up in criminal activity as a result of an addiction, our criminal justice system most often treats them the same as any other criminal. Mental health courts are doing some great work within our province to overcome this problem; however, we need more judges and lawyers and courts to handle the case load to ensure the safety of these individuals and the community at large.

A wise man once said that you can tell how much a society or civilization has grown by the manner in which it treats its criminals. I wonder how this wise man would grade the Province of Newfoundland and Labrador?

Some of the mentally ill individuals we have worked with at Turnings have committed very serious crimes. Some of these crimes were of a sexual nature such as violent rape against children and women of various ages. Frequently we get asked, "How in God's name can you work with these people?" We don't expect anybody who is not involved in our line of work to readily know the answer to this question. However, the answer can be found somewhere within the areas of safety and compassion. If we as a society don't offer support to a person who has served his time in prison for one of the worst crimes imaginable, then that individual will go underground and relocate someplace where he is not known. Being mentally ill and unable to cope with the stresses and challenges of normal society, he will most often re-offend, if for no other reason than to return to prison where he can fit in with others who are the same as him. The result is that one or more people are scarred for life, or worse, and the safety of the community is compromised. Some of these types of individuals we have worked with are more childlike than you could ever imagine and were sexually abused themselves when they were children. I guess what I'm trying to say here is that some of them are not monsters, but little children trapped in a mentally ill adult body. These individuals, in particular, need to be cared for and supported all the days of their lives for their own safety and the safety of innocent women and children, in particular, and the community as a whole.

The stigma associated with mental illness takes on a whole new meaning when you're talking about an offender or ex-offender who has committed violent and hateful crimes.

However, mental illness is just that; it's a very serious illness that can happen to anyone at anytime for a variety of reasons. Why, in God's name, would we not want to help an individual with such a serious illness? At Turnings we feel that not enough is being done to assist individuals with one or more forms of mental illness, and we place special emphasis on individuals of this nature who are presently involved with the criminal justice system.

I hope that our concerns for those with mental health issues don't continue to fall on deaf ears. Maybe this time they'll get it right!

LIVING IN THE IN-BETWEEN

Derrick Pittman, Gander, NL

> "When the adult gives up hope in his ability to cope
> and sees himself incapable of fleeing or fighting, he is
> reduced to a state of depression."
> Ernest Becker, *The Denial of Death*

Depression is a spectre that has been haunting me most of my life. The seeds of the "invisible beast" were planted in childhood and now have come to full bloom in my adult life. If I think back over my life I can see that mental illness has been a constant companion, sometimes lurking on the fringe, sometimes piercing the core of my existence.

I've heard depression described as darkness, the noonday demon, madness, and insanity. I describe it as being wrapped in a cocoon of cold misery. Even this doesn't get at the essence of what it feels like to wake up each morning and feel the dark cloud hovering. It is a disease of doubt. I doubt my thoughts, my emotions, my relationships and I face the "frightening realities of existence, of being alone and doubting my place in the world."

I will give a brief sketch of my life to place things in a certain perspective. I grew up in Labrador City, the youngest of six children. My days were filled with road hockey, softball games, and trips to the cabin on the weekend. I had a normal, even idyllic life. Dad coached hockey and Mom cheered us on in the stands. I can still hear her voice echoing throughout the frozen arena on Saturday mornings. I did well in school, had lots of friends. Everything was going along as planned. I graduated and planned to go to university. After the sun of my childhood there was work to be done.

The first real sign of what would become full-blown social phobia happened one night in the theatre in Labrador City. I felt a strange sensation come over me. I became very nervous, almost paralyzed. This was the genesis of my anxiety and phobia. It burrowed its way into my brain and remained there. I managed to complete my university degree despite not being able to sit through class very often. When I did go, I couldn't speak or even move. I would sit in the same seat in each class, always by the wall and close to the door.

I began my Bachelor of Education program at Memorial University in the fall of 1991, completing my internship in Harlow, England, in December of the following year. By that time my social phobia and panic attacks had subsided somewhat. I was able to stand in front of a class of students without shaking and sweating.

A dark period began in 1993. I had graduated but was unable to find a teaching position. I was twenty-seven, unemployed and living at home with my parents. With each passing day, I sank deeper into a hopeless and helpless void. I had been seeing a psychologist sporadically for a number of years by this time. I was referred to a psychiatric day hospital. It was during this time that I first contemplated suicide. I had a vague plan of taking my white pills and a bottle of vodka to Pippy Park and ending my life. I had been experimenting with taking more than the prescribed dosage of my pills, resulting in losing huge chunks of time from my memory.

Time passed and I was finally offered a teaching position in Davis Inlet in September 1994. I taught there for five years, followed by five years in Sheshatshiu before transferring to Goose Bay. During this time, while still suffering from anxiety and depression, I was able to function as a teacher. I married in 1999 and we had two children.

As a teacher and a father my anxiety increased, which brought on more serious bouts of depression. At one point I finally succumbed to the illness and took six weeks of sick leave. It was at this time that the idea of the stigma of mental illness became very real for me. Stigma is defined as a mark of disgrace. Did I feel ashamed of my illness despite what I knew about it? I confess that I did. In my own way I was creating and perpetuating the stigma by viewing mental illness as somehow different from other diseases. At first I didn't tell my principal why I was off work. Instead I used cryptic phrases to explain my absence from my job. I was afraid to leave my house in case anyone saw me. I didn't look sick, so why was I not at work? How could I explain my illness to someone who saw me? I remember a funny incident one day when I did venture out to go snowshoeing. I heard a snowmobile coming toward me. I dashed off into the woods to hide behind a tree so I wouldn't be recognized. When I thought about this afterwards I had a good chuckle.

I eventually returned to finish the school year and looked forward to the coming September, determined to perform once again as a teacher. I made it until December, when I broke down at work and was hospitalized for eight days. That was the last time I stepped inside a classroom.

Subsequently, I was sent to a psychiatric rehabilitation facility in Ontario for an eight-week program. While there, I had the opportunity to meet and talk with others suffering from a variety of mental illnesses. It helped to be able to talk and not to be judged. I learned about the social, physical, psychological, and spiritual facets of my illness. I learned that there are many ways to take care of myself.

Mental illness has affected my wife and children. My wife struggles to understand as I struggle to explain. I tell my kids that "sometimes Daddy gets sad." I desperately want them to know that it is not their fault. I worry that I will pass on this disease either genetically or environmentally.

Someone once said that the only true philosophical question is whether or not to commit suicide. Philosophy aside, I have been haunted by suicidal thoughts and actions. It is disturbing to think that I could end my own existence. One morning this past April I was pouring some Frosted Flakes for my six-year-old. Suddenly, I was downing a potentially lethal dose of my new medication. Just like that. I told my wife what I had done and she called the ambulance. I was rushed to the hospital where I had my stomach pumped. I was then transferred to the locked psychiatric ward at the Grand Falls hospital.

Earlier, I mentioned the stigma that is attached to mental illness. I guess there are many reasons for this. Perhaps some pop culture influences have been detrimental to the cause of education and awareness of mental illness. Perhaps diseases of the mind make people uncomfortable because they can alter thoughts, emotions and behaviours. I admit I am still nervous about telling people that I suffer from depression. In this way I am guilty of stigmatizing myself and others. Depending on the nature of the relationship, I will tell certain people certain things about my condition. It's not as if people go around telling each other about their medical conditions. I will explain that I am on disability from my career. Or I will say I am a stay-at-home Dad. I don't need to explain my medical condition to everyone I meet.

So what about hope and recovery? My psychiatrist says I am in a battle against darkness. I like this description. We have tried numerous medications (antidepressants, antipsychotics, and anti-anxiety meds) in an effort to stabilize my moods and lift the dark veil a little. I also see a psychologist once a week. We talk about practical matters, like how I can change the way I think about myself and life in general.

I often wonder about the why of my depression. I have thought through this illness a thousand times in search of the ultimate answer. Often I am left with the disturbing fact that I may never know why I have depression. It could be genetic, environmental, brain chemistry or some combination of these. In the end, perhaps it doesn't matter what the answer is. The reality is that I have to learn to live with this mental illness.

I feel like a ghost in my own life. A friend of mine who has experienced mental illness calls it a tortured existence. I want to come back to life. I want to see my kids graduate from school and become healthy, happy adults. I want to grow old with my wife and spoil our grandchildren.

Ultimately, depression is a battle with myself. I am constantly trying to understand, to redeem myself, to change myself. I live in a middle world between accepting who I am and changing who I am.

FIXING THE MUSIC

Rosalind Wiseman, Mount Pearl, NL

I was six years old. The warm fog hung over my bright blonde curls. Crouched on the top step in front of my house, I opened a faded pink box. A hint of sparkles on one corner remained. The plastic ballerina popped up not so gracefully and a song started to play. As I held the music box up to my ear I heard the plinking of music notes. My curiosity got the best of me. I slowly pried apart the box and found a small metal box inside. I still, however, couldn't see or understand how it worked. How did all these parts go together to play me a song? I decided to use a butter knife to break it open. This revealed a wheel with Braille-like markings and a fork-like metal arm that scraped over the bumps to make that plinking sound. What a disappointment. A mix of guilt and humiliation swept over me. What had I expected? Tiny beings playing tiny instruments inside my music box? Why couldn't I just be happy with hearing the music? Sometimes things are better left to the imagination. Sometimes we need to dig deeper in order to learn about ourselves and the world. Sadly, sometimes we tear ourselves apart to try and understand how we work. To find where our music comes from or often why it went away.

When I turned sixteen I was still full of wonder. I worked hard all summer so I could buy my own school clothes. What a treat to have clothes from the mall and not the Sears catalogue. That September I wore bright, funky clothes and I loved them.

The colours, however, soon turned dark. I had worked very hard that summer: a community clean-up student project during the day, babysitting a couple of hours each evening, and a couple of over-nights here and there filling in my grandmother's home care. She had Alzheimer's disease. I tried so hard to understand what was happening to her. My mind was very tired. I was a very busy girl. You would think that I would sleep solid at night. So why was I still so energetic most of the time? So energetic that I agitated myself. Did I not need sleep anymore? It seemed not. I would laugh and joke my way through the school day, get easily annoyed with family members at home, and cry at night. I would wander to my parents' room after hours of lying awake and ask my mom if she could come sleep in my bed. So being the great mom she was and is, she did. And many more dark nights since then when I was ill.

It didn't take me very long to know something was very wrong with me. Especially when it got to the point that I told a couple of my friends in school to tell others I had laryngitis. I couldn't have a conversation. My mind was so jumbled. Like a frantic hungry sea-gull — thoughts seemed to swoop down just long enough for me to start to speak and quickly fly away again leaving me frustrated and speechless. I couldn't even finish a yawn or a sneeze let alone a thought or a sentence. At times my eyes continuously blinked. My perception was scrambled as well. When I tried to concentrate on a class discussion it seemed either nothing made any sense, or worse, everything had "special meaning" to me. Times like these, everything a teacher would speak about I had a memory in life to go along with it. Every description brought up a clear image in my mind and then an emotion. I was very sensitive. It felt like I was in tune with everyone's feelings too. I interpreted every glance, every cough, every whisper. Sounds which normally would go unnoticed were now all I could take in. My senses were heightened. I remember in one of my classes spinning around in my seat and saying to a girl: "Is it just me or is everyone acting strange today?" She answered sweetly: "No, I think it's just you." Of course then I thought she was acting strange too.

That specific school day ended with me sitting in front of the principal in her office. To her credit I have to say she pretty quickly determined that I was ill. She saw the look in my eyes when half my sentence went away and I couldn't find it. I agreed with her and told her I knew I wasn't well and had already set up a doctor's appointment for that day. That was actually the truth. My sister was in nursing school and when I first started feeling "sick" I tried to find a condition in one of her books that would explain my symptoms. I decided I was malnourished and my brain was deprived of vital nutrients. I figured the doctor would tell me what to do to fix it and I would soon be all better. A few vitamins maybe. Of course to his credit he knew of my family history of bipolar illness (though I did not) and sent me to a hospital in the big city. Coming from a community of about three hundred people, that was a stay I'll never forget.

The doctor sent me in a car with my father to go home, get clothes and then go to the hospital. Very bad idea. I tried to get out of the car while it was moving. Not trying to hurt myself. Just desperately trying to escape. Keep in mind: I thought I was misdiagnosed and now they were going to lock me up in a mental institution. I just needed some vitamins for God's sake! When you're sick, your truth and your perception is your reality. Your fears are very real. I managed to get out of his car and quickly got in with some tourists who promptly and nervously brought me to the police station under my direction. My shirt was all torn from poor Dad trying to keep me in the car. The police would not release me to him even though he had a letter from the doctor. They believed my intense terror over the letter that my father held out in his shaking hand. The police escorted me back to the doctor's office, where I received a shot in my behind. I woke up a few days later, with debilitating muscle cramps that caused me to faint and fall in front of the nursing station. It seemed the hospital kept giving me what the doctor had given me in his office that evening to knock me out. It was called Haldol and was no longer necessary. So what did they do? Pile my lanky teenage body into a wheelchair, give me another shot of that same drug . . . and while I drifted off into a haze I remember a song going through my head that my mom taught me when I was about four years old. It was the theme song from the *Friendly Giant*: "Early one morning just as the sun was shining I heard a maid sing in the valley below. Oh don't deceive me, oh never leave me, how could you treat a poor maiden so?" Oh to be sixteen again. No thank you.

Just think for a second how people perceive things. For instance: A well person walks out her front door in the morning to go to work. The sky is darkening in the peaceful early silence. She pauses for a moment, then runs back into her house to get her umbrella because she believes it might rain. An unwell person walks out her front door in the morning to go to work. The sky is darkening in the intense morning silence. She is paralyzed for a moment with fear, then runs back into her house because she believes this is a sign that something bad will happen today.

I was discharged from hospital after one month and was stabilized on Lithium. As soon as possible I weaned myself off it. I lasted somehow for ten years without it. Looking back it was like the longest and slowest roller-coaster ride you would never want to take. I managed, however, to get by until my graduating year in university. I always took on so much at once. Too many jobs, too many classes and too many drinks in my downtime eventually caught up with me. I was hospitalized in Halifax for a month. This time I was put on Epival, an anti-convulsive medicine which made me extremely sensitive to light and so very ill. Soon after being discharged from hospital I stopped taking my medication. On the bright side, during my hospital stay I was able to complete the necessary school work to graduate with my class.

I lasted for a couple more years until I was hospitalized in St. John's again. I knew I was very sick that last time and my poor mother was trying so hard to take care of me. I just couldn't do that to her anymore. I checked myself into the hospital and started taking Lithium again. This time I kept taking it. That was about three and a half years ago. I am now happily married with a beautiful baby girl. I did not take Lithium while I was pregnant. I know, however, that just because I was okay while off my medication, that doesn't mean I don't need it. Rock climbers could safely climb many times without a safety harness too, but I wouldn't suggest it. It's not worth it. Why take the chance? Lithium doesn't make me feel ill at all. It gives me the safety harness I need to go where I need to go in life.

It took me a long time to learn to take care of myself. It's a daily choice to be as healthy as I can be. People like me need professional help. Let's face it, sometimes the help we get is far from professional or even helpful for that matter. It's often a blanket treatment for all who fall within a category. I've lived in fear of some scarier hospital workers than Steven King could imagine, and they really do exist. We, of course, are individuals with different barriers to wellness. We are whole people, with dreams and knowledge and heart. We help each other and many of us have suffered in silence for many years. I have been an advocate for mental health consumers long before I even knew what an advocate was. I was raised to treat people how I would like to be treated. We are all more alike than different. Whether we live with mental illness or live to help those with mental illness. I dream to do both. And I go through my life as most people do. Doctors and patients alike. We try to learn from our mistakes and move towards our goals. Accepting help along the way from those who care.

I live a stable life now. I work full-time. Right now I am on maternity leave. My husband and I take good care of each other. He understands that I live with bipolar illness and he loves me anyway. He sees the complete person that I am. There are many things that I am. Only one of them is my illness. Now I think a lot about how and when I will explain my illness to my daughter. I'm hoping she will love me anyway too.

MY SISTER, SHEILA RUTH KENT

Eileen Kavanagh, Conception Bay South, NL

My sister Sheila was buried on October 13, 2007. One might have considered that an unlucky day. For Sheila it was a happy day.

Let me tell you our story.

Sheila Ruth, the second daughter of Jack and Rhoda Kent, was born on Bell Island, March 19, 1944. Because she was born during Sheila's Brush, the storm we always get in March, she brought her name with her. Sheila was a bright, beautiful girl who did well academically and socially. She had always wanted to be a nurse but after high school graduation was still too young to enter nurse's training so she found other employment until she was old enough to follow her dream. She trained at St. Clare's Mercy Hospital, graduated and successfully passed the dreaded R.N. certification. She worked at St. Clare's until she married a young teacher from Red Island and went off to Ontario. She was immediately hired at Scarborough General Hospital where she worked in intensive care.

Her first pregnancy was uneventful but after her daughter was born she suffered what everyone thought was postpartum depression. Problems persisted and she was diagnosed with schizophrenia. She had several bouts where she ended up in a psychiatric hospital where her treatment included electric shock therapy. This was 1967 and she was devastated and embarrassed by this diagnosis. Eventually her diagnosis was changed to manic-depression. She was still just as sick but she liked this diagnosis better as there was somewhat less of a stigma attached.

Against the suggestion of her psychiatrist she again became pregnant. After this baby the episodes became more frequent and lasted longer. Juggling a career with shift work, two children, a mental health problem and the meds was just too much for her so she resigned her job. Her marriage, her mental health and her self-esteem all deteriorated. She was becoming more and more withdrawn, socializing only with immediate family.

Around 1990 she decided to move to Cambridge where I was living. Her daughter was finished university and not living at home, her son was just starting university in another town, and her husband was remarried so she really had no reason not to move. I realized this would be extra responsibility for me but thought with a new start she'd do better. I was wrong.

I read everything I could about manic-depression, talked to her previous psychiatrist and went with her for the first appointment with the new psychiatrist in Cambridge. I felt she was off to a good start and tried to keep her active, hoping activity would prevent more trips to the hospital but it was too late. Her inability to function in a society that did not understand mental illness had eaten up all her self-esteem and she didn't trust herself in public anymore. She just stayed home smoking cigarettes, avoiding almost all social situations.

Sheila and I struggled through her breakdowns. She would hallucinate or become very paranoid suspecting the neighbours of all kinds of transgressions. She would call me at all hours of the night to check that I was okay or to express concern about some other family member. She frequently called the fire department, claiming she smelled gas or smoke. She would call the police about imagined burglars. Yet it was so difficult to get her into the hospital. She would never go on her own and had to be a threat to herself or someone else before the psychiatrist would sign her in. I worried so much for her safety but had to wait until someone else called the police before they would admit her into hospital. Then she would be there for three to six weeks. I still think if she could have been admitted sooner it would not have been so severe. Laws made to protect sometimes do the opposite. Perhaps if there weren't so many stigmas with this illness she might have been more open to going sooner.

This was very traumatic for both of us. Can you imagine watching your intelligent sister agonizing because she sees bugs all over her house and her skin? Can you see yourself stand by helpless as your sister, trying to kill imagined bugs, washes in bleach until her skin is all cracked and bleeding? Can you imagine seeing the police take your sister in handcuffs, in the snow, in her slippers, just because she's sick? These are just some of the images that will be with me forever.

Can you imagine the grief and fear she felt when she saw herself as a misfit (that's her exact word), when she believed everyone was against her, laughing at and talking about her, when there were little men hiding outside her house, when people's faces became distorted, when there were bugs running all over her, when her phone lines were tapped, when her money, her underwear, her cigarettes, were all missing? These things only happened in her mind but *to her they were very real.*

Can you imagine being restrained in a straitjacket, locked in a room or on a psychiatric ward, or facing shock treatment? Add to that the stigma attached to your illness. It's easy to say, "I have asthma," or "I have diabetes," but it's not so easy to say, "I have a personality disorder." How many people have said to you, "My sister is bipolar," or "My brother is schizophrenic"? It's very much in the closet. People normally come home from hospital and share their funny hospital stories, but people coming home from a psychiatric hospital won't share their stories and they have some real stories to share. Sheila was so embarrassed about being in a psychiatric hospital that she always manufactured a physical ailment as an excuse for being there. Just admitting she was in hospital was too painful for her.

She continued to have bouts of illness, ending up in the psychiatric hospital. Any change in routine would make her sick. Once she came to Newfoundland for a holiday and ended up in the Waterford Hospital for several weeks. Even a simple cold would throw her out of balance. Her doctors frequently changed her meds and tried new ones but nothing seemed to work for very long. Eventually her diagnosis was changed to schizo-affective disorder.

In 2004, when I moved back to Newfoundland, it was with a heavy heart that I left Sheila in a retirement home in Cambridge. All her care was provided and a nurse administered her meds. Another sister and I debated moving her here but she was very happy where she was and wanted to stay close to her two children. I talked to her almost every day and went back four times a year to visit her.

The ACT Team was in place at this time. This team consisted of a psychiatrist, nurses, and social workers. This wonderful team treated Sheila with respect and was an immense support to Sheila and me. I am very grateful for their help.

She was a heavy smoker and developed a bad cough that had been treated with several doses of antibiotics but never really went away. One night in September she called to tell me she was very sick. She was wheezing and having trouble breathing. I called the nurse at the home who told me the doctor said she couldn't do any more and that they thought it was psychosomatic. They had done x-rays and nothing showed up.

A nurse from the ACT Team took her to the hospital the next morning where she was diagnosed with mental health issues and sent to London Psych. She called me from the psychiatric hospital and she sounded terrible. I really did not know if this was real or imagined because sometimes she had trouble with reality and I wasn't there to see for myself. Finally she called and said a new x-ray showed a mass in her lung. She often said things like this so I called the hospital to check and the nurse I talked to confirmed it to be true. Then her daughter called to say that she had been called in and it was serious. My sister and I left Newfoundland to go and visit her.

The whole family was there and Sheila was very happy.

We stayed in London overnight and went to the cancer doctor with her in the morning. He was talking about a biopsy but figured from the x-rays that she had a rapid lung cancer. Sheila was calm and rational and was very sure she did not want a biopsy or any other treatment. She was moved back to Cambridge hospital where I noticed marked improvement in her self-esteem. She was calling the shots now and she was amazing. She decided her treatment prior to and following her death. Although she died within days, she had appeared so much better that even the hospital staff were amazed and thought perhaps the diagnosis was incorrect.

She and I talked right up until she lost consciousness a few hours before she died. She talked about how much she had suffered through her mental illness, how she didn't fit in anywhere and how she knew she would soon be at peace. She wrote me a lovely note thanking me for "rescuing" her so often. She thanked other family members, the ACT Team, and her favourite nurses at the retirement home. She was more in control of her life then than she had been for years. She was physically sick now and knew this cancer would soon kill her but she could deal with that. She was in hospital and she was dying, but this sickness, this trip to the hospital, had no stigma attached. *It was easier to be in a regular bed dying of cancer than to be on the psych ward or in a psychiatric hospital being treated for mental illness. Cancer had no stigma.*

Sheila died a very peaceful death and is resting in a beautiful cemetery near the homes of her children. I will tell her story to anyone who will listen because I believe the immense sadness her mental illness caused her would have been greatly lessened if there were no stigma attached. We need to take mental illness out of the closet and accept it as openly as we do physical illness. Only by talking about it and educating people will we remove the stigma. Once, when Sheila was sick, I mentioned in the staff-room at work that I was worried about her and why I was worried. The silence was deafening as people processed what I had just said. Then another staff member said, "My brother is schizophrenic," and she shared some information about him. Gradually others shared privately or in the staff-room about their own, or family members', mental health issues, with one staff member openly discussing her own bipolar disorder. People actually seemed relieved to be able to discuss it openly and I've since discovered that every family has members with mental health issues. There is no shame in that and we need to stop attaching shame to it. It's too late for my sister Sheila, but it's not too late for the next generation, for my grandchildren, Sheila's grandchildren or your grandchildren, some of whom are sure to have to face mental health issues in their own lives.

I miss my sister Sheila. She was one of the kindest, most thoughtful people I've ever known. She was also the saddest. I believe she has finally found peace.

REFLECTIONS ON MENTAL HEALTH:
ACCEPTANCE OF ILLNESS DOESN'T COME EASILY

Geoff Chaulk, St. John's, NL

Excerpted and updated from an article published in The Telegram, *May 2006.*

In August 2005, I had the difficult experience of taking sick leave from my job due to what became my worst bout of depression. I was then the executive director of the Canadian Mental Health Association in the province. I was originally treated for depression in my early twenties. I am now fifty-one and have been treated several times since. I should note that, as a teenager, I made an attempt at suicide, an attempt significant enough to greatly upset my family and to be referred to a psychiatrist at the Janeway hospital. For most people who live with mental illness, onset generally takes place in late adolescence or early adulthood. As an adult, treatment for me has involved a combination of medication, psychotherapy and self-help.

Over the years, I have become more accepting of my illness, but this acceptance has not come easily and, in some respects, it is still not complete. Also, I am someone who has spent his professional life, close to thirty years, working in the area of mental health. I wanted to write about my recent experience as part of my own process of acceptance and to share with others a message that is hopeful. For me, when dealing with episodes of depression, the signs of onset are not always clear. However, the one sign I am unable to deny is sleep disturbance. When my sleep is disturbed for a period of time, and not just a night or two, I grow concerned that I may be becoming depressed. Sleep disturbance struck again the spring of 2005.

This, in itself, was unusual for me as I find summer a time when generally I don't worry about becoming depressed. With the passing of days and weeks, I realized that my concentration was poor (I read a lot and found that I could not follow a plot line), my appetite dropped off as did some weight and, of course, my mood was depressed. I also had rather catastrophic emotional reactions (in my head and not shared with anyone) to relatively minor issues work-related and otherwise. Anxiety plagued me and would erupt for no apparent reason.

It is in my current healthy state of mind that I can look back on those months and see more clearly what I was like. You will notice that some of the symptoms that I experience are physical in nature. This is not unusual for many people who live with depression. Also, and I'm a bit embarrassed to admit this, but as the signs and symptoms started to set in, I abruptly stopped my antidepressant medication. I think I was frustrated and angry that even with medication (albeit a fairly mild one), I was getting ill again. If you are reading this and taking antidepressant medication, I strongly suggest you not do what I did unless you have discussed it with your physician. There is evidence that people should be tapered off antidepressant medication so as to avoid withdrawal-like symptoms.

Having suffered through a couple of summer months being fairly sleep-deprived and feeling worse over time, and following a discussion with a colleague, I finally made an appointment with my family doctor. He is a great guy who seemed to know rather quickly that I was depressed. He was prescribing the antidepressant medication I had been taking. He was kind and generous with his time that morning in August and he gently told me I would need to stay off work. He also wanted me referred to a psychiatrist for an opinion on medication change and psychotherapy support. I'm fortunate to have a family doctor, and a good one at that. For most Canadians, it is a family doctor they reach out to when experiencing the signs and symptoms of depression. I was eventually referred to a fine psychiatrist who took the most detailed history on my mental health and mental illness that I have experienced in more than twenty-five years of periodic treatment.

As a result of this assessment, my medication was changed with good results, my mood went back to normal, my appetite returned and eventually my sleep pattern became healthy again. Medication is an important part of my recovery, but it is not the only part. I have great support from my family and close friends. Even neighbours in the apartment building where I live reached out to me. I continued with self-help and I am in the process of restoring my spiritual life.

Good mental health should never be taken for granted. Twenty per cent of Canadians will experience a mental illness in his or her lifetime and eight per cent will experience depression. In a recent study, twenty per cent of women surveyed in the workplace showed signs and symptoms of depression. More than fifty per cent of Canadians identify work as the most significant source of stress in their lives. Stress that is not addressed can lead to physical and mental health problems.

Trust me, losing your mental health is a very painful experience. Recovery is possible and many of us have recovered, continue to recover and are moving forward with our lives.

INDEX

MENTAL HEALTH ORGANIZATIONS & RESOURCES

Canadian Mental Health Association, Newfoundland and Labrador Division (CMHA-NL)
70 the Boulevard, 1ˢᵗ Floor
St. John's, NL A1A 1K2
Tel: (709) 753-8550, Toll free 1-877-753-8550
Fax: (709) 753-8537
Email: office@cmhanl.ca
Website: www.cmhanl.ca

CHANNAL (Consumers' Health Awareness Network of Newfoundland and Labrador)
Tel: (709) 636-4709, Toll Free 1-888-636-4709
Fax: (709) 635-4688
Executive Director: ed@channal.ca
Provincial Volunteer Coordinator: vol@channal.ca
Website: www.channal.ca

Community Mental Health Initiative (CMHI)
63 Broadway, PO Box 2006
Corner Brook, NL A2H 6J8
Tel: (709) 634-4117
Fax: (709) 634-4155
Email: cmhi.nl@gmail.com
Website: www.envision.ca/webs/cmhi

Eating Disorder Foundation of Newfoundland and Labrador
31 Peet Street, Suite 208
St. John's, NL A1B 3W8
Tel: (709) 722-0500
Fax: (709) 722-0552
Email: info@edfnl.ca
Website: www.edfnl.ca

Independent Living Resource Centre (ILRC)
4 Escasoni Place
St. John's, NL A1C 3R6
Tel: (709) 722-4031
Fax: (709) 722-0147
TTY: (709) 722-7998
Toll Free: 1-866-722-4031
Email: info@ilrc-nl.ca
Website: www.ilrc-nl.ca

Mental Health Crisis Line
In St. John's: 737-4668
Toll Free: 1-888-737-4668

The Pottle Centre
323 Hamilton Avenue
St. John's, NL A1E 1K1
Tel: (709) 753-2143
Website: www.thepottlecentre.com

Schizophrenia Society of Newfoundland and Labrador
205-206WB Waterford Hospital
Waterford Bridge Road
St. John's, NL A1E 4J8
Tel: (709) 777-3335
Fax: (709) 777-3524
Email: ssnl1@yahoo.ca
Website: http://www.ssnl.org/

Stella Burry Community Services
142 Military Road
St. John's, NL A1C 2E6
Tel: (709) 738-7805
Fax: (709) 738-1030
Email: info@stellaburry.ca
Website: www.stellaburry.ca

Department of Health and Community Services, Government of Newfoundland and Labrador:
Website: www.health.gov.nl.ca

Newfoundland and Labrador Regional Health Authorities:
Website: www.easternhealth.ca
Website: www.westernhealth.nl.ca
Website: www.centralhealth.nl.ca
Website: www.lghealth.ca

CPSIA information can be obtained at www.ICGtesting.com
Printed in the USA
LVOW01s2359050503314

376248LV00011B/271/P